DEATH CAN WAIT

Stories from Cancer Survivors

By

Frank Hegyi
Roslyn Franken
Jacquelin Holzman
Max Keeping

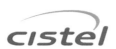

*Partial financial support for the project
was provided by Cistel Foundation*

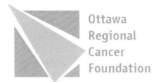

Ottawa
Regional
Cancer
Foundation

*All profits from the sales of this book will be donated,
through the Ottawa Regional Cancer Foundation,
to support cancer research and the facilities
which provide treatment for cancer patients.*

http://www.ottawacancer.ca/

Published by:

Baico Publishing
102-C McEwen Ave.
Ottawa, Ontario K2B 5K7
Tel: (613) 829-5141
www.baico.ca
E-mail: baico@bellnet.ca

Printed by Documents Majemta Inc.

WHAT CANCER CANNOT DO

Cancer is limited:

It cannot cripple love

It cannot shatter hope

It cannot corrode faith

It cannot destroy peace

It cannot kill friendship

It cannot suppress memories

It cannot silence courage

It cannot invade the soul

It cannot steal eternal life

It cannot conquer the Spirit

Author unknown

———————■———————

INTRODUCTION

—————————■—————————

The quartet who have put together this book, Frank Hegyi, Roslyn Franken, Jacquelin Holzman, and Max Keeping, all share a trait in common - the desire, and the ability, to transcend their own personal circumstance and to thereby help others.

They have battled cancer, and as soldiers in this struggle, they have come together to offer help of a most vital sort. Facts and details about cancer in its many forms are readily available. What is not that available is true, unvarnished insight into what goes on behind the scenes, behind the outer facade.

What goes through peoples' minds when they get the shattering news? What feelings and emotions do they wrestle with as they cling onto life? What attitudes are helpful, what attitudes are destructive?

This is a book that addresses these issues. Every single contributor has his or her own unique story, a story they share with the world. It takes courage and precision to be able to share, to reveal what really goes on. We are so grateful to those who have shared in this profound manner.

This is so important for those who unfortunately are destined to be told they have cancer, a steadily rising number of between one-third and one-half of the population. No two cancers are alike, no two individuals are alike. But we all share a common desire to live, to be healthy, and to have the necessary wherewithal to surmount life-threatening crises.

This book provides so much of that in a personal, even intimate way. The battle against cancer is being fought on so many fronts - research, treatment, prevention, etc. The emotional side cannot be ignored. This is a book written with feeling, about feelings in times of gigantic challenge. May it enure to everyone feeling better.

Rabbi Reuven P. Bulka

ABOUT THE BOOK

—■—

All contributors of this book are cancer survivors. We believe that cancer can be beaten. Early diagnosis, effective medical treatments, diets and healthy lifestyle are all important elements for surviving cancer. Those of us who travelled the road to recovery have found that positive attitude at the time of diagnosis and during treatments was also an important element of survival. Hence, we want to share our stories with newly diagnosed patients in an effort to provide moral support while they are fighting their courageous battles.

These stories provide an insight into the incredible courage of some of the people who have received the news which initially appeared to be a death sentence. Others have treated the news as a wakeup call to make changes in their lifestyles. Then there are stories of emotional crisis and the challenges of surviving this dreaded disease.

We have also compiled information about the major cancer types to serve as a reference material for newly diagnosed cancer patients, their families, friends and co-workers. In the foot notes, linkages are provided to internet web sites which contain more detailed description of the different cancer types and their associated symptoms. These symptoms should be treated only as an incentive to seek medical advice, especially because early diagnosis is one of the most important ingredients of beating the big "C".

THE STORIES

Diane

Non-Hodgkin's Lymphoma

Halloween, 2005

———————■———————

A monster came knocking at my door and it wasn't in the form of a child dressed in a cute costume; it was in the form of cancer. I was diagnosed with Non-Hodgkin's Lymphoma. I was shocked and devastated as well as afraid. This was the same disease my mother had battled and lost 16 years ago. Now I was faced with the same battle. I had just turned fifty that summer and looking forward to the next decade which would herald in my retirement, my children's graduations from University, their growing up and leaving home and a whole bunch of travelling plans. I was now faced with mortality; something that I wasn't expecting to face so soon. Life does not stop and demands attention so basically my husband and I went home and handed out candies to the trick or treaters and started to formulate cancer into our lives. I have no idea how I got through the next weeks anxiously waiting for the medical system to kick in. My husband was the rock I clung to and the calming effect I sought when I was distraught. Keeping myself busy at work and with everyday living took my mind off the days ahead and what they would bring.

Surgery was performed to excise a tumour for further investigation to determine the treatment course and a CT scan was performed. One very anxious day while waiting for the call that would introduce me to my oncologist I came home from work to greet my husband, screaming at the top of my lungs "I WANT MY LIFE BACK". At that moment I acknowledged that my life was never going to be the same again. It hadn't changed outworldly. I was still living my life as I had before the diagnosis, but inside me life was altered. I had to learn to deal with and live in this altered state. Everyone has an inner strength to deal with disasters in their own way and time. I found strength and support in continuing to conduct my life the same way I had always done. Busying myself with work and family helped me cope with my anxiety. My husband's belief in my strength and his constant calming effect on me when I was in states of anxiety was my life line at the time of diagnosis, through treatment and is still to this day.

Initially a diagnosis of cancer changed my outlook on life in that I realized how precious my life was to me. It forced me to realize that my life is not infinite and it has forced me to see it as finite. I appreciate the little things in my life, spending more time revelling in parts of my life I had no time for before cancer. This outlook has been more difficult to maintain though, as one tends to get sucked back into the daily flow of life; the house needs cleaning, the kids need chauffeuring, the bills need paying and on it goes. Life goes on around you; it doesn't stop with a diagnosis of cancer. I had to learn to put myself first. Easier said than done.

My lifestyle has not drastically changed since being diagnosed. I felt what I was doing before cancer was good for me. Eating, sleeping, and exercising well were part of my lifestyle, which I have continued to maintain with one addition, I am taking more time for myself, spending more time pampering myself, finding time to do the things I want to do and not allowing anything stressful to bother me.

The major impact cancer has had on my life is that I am not putting off tomorrow what I can do today. I am not waiting for retirement or the right time to achieve my goals and live my plans. I am making my dreams happen now and I am enjoying every minute!

So the diagnosis was cancer. What next? Dealing with the medical system for treatment. Next to the fear of a diagnosis of cancer was the fear of having to deal with the medical system. Long wait times were the worst. Waiting for surgery, waiting for CT scans, waiting to see the oncologist and waiting for treatment to begin. All I wanted at this stage was to get on with the treatment. The waiting was something I had no control over and it was causing much anxiety. Treatment couldn't come soon enough for me. The cancer was aggressive and it had taken a good foot hold by the time I was diagnosed. The biopsy of the lymph nodes and the CT and MRI scans had proven this. Once I had the pathology report in my hands I started researching the disease in detail and how it pertained to me. There were many details I had to force myself to read. Some gave me hope, others put me in despair. But I needed to be prepared for my appointment with the doctor. The appointment day had finally come and I was armed with much information. Information is power and it was for me that day. The treatment he suggested was the one I had researched, the information he gave me was familiar. I was able to ask questions intelligently. All this had made me feel in control and safe. Treatment started within two days. The waiting had ended. I had to put my trust in God and the system treating me. The research I had done before treatment was a great asset in allowing me to trust the doctor's choice of treatment. My fears of dealing with the medical system were diminishing with each treatment I received through those ten months. I was well taken care of and I was responding with no major adverse reactions or events. This is all I could ask for at the time. Knowledge has helped me come to terms with my disease. I felt more in control and it has given me an abundance of hope. I have come from thoughts of my cancer as a death sentence to one of being a chronic disease that can be managed. Two and half years later I continue to amass information, everything that will help me live well with cancer. I am alive and well, continuing to make my plans reality and enjoying life as it unfolds.

After chemotherapy I received a month of radiation treatment for residual disease in my hip area and four months later was entered into a maintenance Rituxan program for two years, of which I have completed one. I have continued to work since the beginning of my treatment in 2005 and am working towards retirement in another 2 years at the age of 55. I am aiming for a long remission and hope that at least it will stay dormant long enough to enjoy some retirement years with my husband and for science to progress towards a cure. I lived a good life before cancer; diligently taking care of myself so continuing to do this is no hardship. I have incorporated in my diet many foods that have cancer fighting agents and I supplement with vitamin D during the winter months. I exercise faithfully, eat well, and get plenty of quality sleep. Knowing that I am doing everything in my power to keep myself healthy and disease free gives me confidence and hope.

Do I worry about recurrence? All the time. The worry varies in degrees depending on how I am feeling physically and mentally. After treatment every little ailment would send me into worry mode. I have learned to temper this with time but the worry never goes away. I know that when worry of recurrence becomes overwhelming and starts to affect my life I will seek professional help. My mental health plays a major role in my physical health and how I perceive my future living with cancer.

I hope a diagnosis of cancer a second time will be easier to deal with knowing that I have prepared myself mentally and physically to the best of my ability.

Breaking the news of my diagnosis to family, friends and co-workers had to be the most difficult task I have ever been faced with. Dealing with everybody's reaction to the news was no easier.

It made me so sad to have to burden my family and friends with news like this, especially my father who had lived this experience 16 years ago when my mother was diagnosed with the same cancer. I was dreading telling him so much that I delayed it until he was settled in his winter home in Florida. I thought telling him over the phone would be easier for both of us. It wasn't.

I was amazed how everybody at work rallied around me. The generosity of concern, gifts and support from everybody I knew was overwhelming. Knowing that I am loved and supported has helped me the most through the tough times I have experienced in battling this disease and will continue to help me face whatever lays ahead. I could not have gone through what I did without the support of family and friends.

I feel the best way for my relatives, friends and co-workers to interact with me as a newly diagnosed cancer patient, was to treat me as they had always done, with kindness and consideration and with the knowledge that if I needed help in any way I would call upon them.

Elaine Senack

Ottawa, Ontario

Breast Cancer

———————■———————

I always had "lumpy boobs" which is a layman's term for fibrocystic disease, which results in benign breast lumps which come and go. I had discovered a rather persistent lump back in 2005, which was biopsied in January of 2006 with negative results. However, this lump didn't go away and my doctor recommended another biopsy which was done in November, 2006.

I received my diagnosis of breast cancer on December 6th, 2006, at 11 am in the morning via a phone call from the physician who had performed my breast biopsy a week earlier. My first question was to ask him to repeat who was calling as I had totally blocked the event from my memory. My second question was to ask if he was sure he had the right person. I was in total shock and disbelief. I was 56 years old, and for the first time in my life, started to seriously think that I may not have a whole lot of time left in this world.

My husband knew there was something wrong the minute he returned home from work and saw my face. I never was very good at hiding my feelings. We spent the evening and well into the night talking about what this diagnosis might mean, although neither one of us had any idea yet of what lay ahead. However, we both knew that whatever happened, we could deal with it and would deal with it together.

Because Christmas was only 3 weeks away, we mutually decided not to tell our adult sons and daughter-in-laws or the rest of our family until after the holidays. That way, we wouldn't spoil the fun and excitement of Christmas with our kids and grandkids. In retrospect, I think those weeks prior to others knowing of my diagnosis were very hard on my husband. He was extremely strong and supportive for me, but he probably could have used someone's shoulder to lean on. The tentacles of a cancer diagnosis reach far beyond the individual.

The next few weeks were a flurry of doctor appointments, blood work and numerous tests and x-rays. The size of the tumor and spread of the cells into the surrounding tissue meant I would need to have a mastectomy and would not have the option of a lumpectomy or breast reconstruction. The tests were grueling but necessary to determine if the cancer cells had spread to other parts of my body. Some days, the anxiety was crippling. I felt that I had lost control, not only of my body but of my future. The unknown loomed over me like a big grey cloud. I tried to keep a positive attitude and the voice in my head kept telling me over and over, you can deal with this.

I read everything I could get my hands on related to breast cancer. I soon found there is a wealth of information on the Canadian and American Cancer Foundation, Health Canada and the Regional Ottawa Cancer Foundation websites. I also read a book called "Dr. Susan Love's Breast Book" which provides straight forward, factual, up to date information about breast cancer and treatment. I referred to this book many, many times over the course of my diagnosis and treatment.

Even though I have a nursing background, the breadth and depth of information was sometimes overwhelming. So much has changed and continues to change as cancer research provides evidence based improvement in treatment choices and outcomes. The important thing is to be as informed as possible, know and understand your options for treatment and ask questions. Don't assume anything. Personally, I found it much easier to deal with the facts than to deal with the unknown.

Once family, friends and co-workers were aware of my diagnosis and upcoming surgery, I was overwhelmed by the outpouring of support. A former co-worker, who had been diagnosed with breast cancer and undergone chemotherapy and radiation the previous year, telephoned me one morning. She and I chatted for about an hour and she provided me with a wealth of information and support from her own personal experiences. The conversation was very positive and directed towards the support systems in place to alleviate the side effects of treatment to the best place to buy mastectomy bras. Our conversation also made me realize that throughout treatment, I would still be able to continue to carry out my day to day activities, and my anxiety level dropped considerably. I started to think of my diagnosis and impending treatments as a "blip" in the roadmap of my life.

People I had not spoke to in many months were there to lend a hand, drop off food and just call to see how I was doing. The support didn't stop once I had recovered from my surgery. My family and friends were a phenomenal support. It made me realize how much I loved my family and how important friends and family were to me. My family has become much closer and we don't take anything for granted any more.

Chemotherapy treatments started 6 weeks after my mastectomy and I was far more anxious about having chemo then I was about having surgery. Would I be able to cope with the side effects, and the hair loss – yikes! My husband came to all 8 chemo sessions with me, providing emotional support, making sure I was comfortable and getting me something to drink or eat when I needed it. Becoming part of the patient population of the Chemotherapy Unit at The Ottawa Hospital was a humbling experience for both of us. Some of the patients looked so young and some patients looked very ill. However, we seemed to all belong to an inner circle, or secret club, brought together by our medical circumstances. When a patient completed their final chemotherapy treatment, they rang a big bell close to the exit door and the rest of us clapped and cheered when they accomplished this milestone. I could hardly wait to the day when I too, could ring that bell.

25 daily radiation treatments followed chemotherapy and by the end of September, 2007, my treatment was completed.

I continued with my management consulting business, working part time hours and having the flexibility to schedule work and meetings around my treatment schedules. Working provided me with a focus besides my treatments, and kept me visible and part of day to day interactions with my working life. I was also able to attend social and family gatherings throughout the year. Both the professional and social interactions with others provided the mental boost that kept my attitude and outlook positive. I also think being visible helped others overcome their own fears of approaching me and thinking I was cloistered away, suffering from treatment side effects.

Now, a year later, I am feeling well and my energy is back to normal. My husband and I are both much more in tune with each others feelings and make an effort to spend more time together and to spend time with our family.

I have needed to seek physiotherapy for mild lymphedema and loss of full movement in my right arm. However, exercise and aquafit is helping those symptoms and contributing to my overall physical fitness. I still have some lingering side effects from the chemotherapy treatments but they are manageable with medication. I continue to visit my oncologists every 6 months and have no sign of reoccurrence.

My life is good and I live each day to the fullest. I have managed to stop thinking about all the "what ifs" and get on with living. My priorities have changed and quality of life is of the utmost importance to me. Longevity may not be in my future, but no one has a crystal ball to be able to see and know what the future holds. I would rather leave this world knowing that I enjoyed my life and contributed to the happiness of others than to live out my days being miserable and worrying about things I can't control.

What would my advice be to others who are newly diagnosed with cancer?

- Reach out to others. Don't be afraid to ask for help. Others want to help you.

- Tell those you love that you love them.

- Enjoy life's little moments, like a sunset, a drive in the country, and the hugs from your grandchildren.

- Be an informed consumer. By that, I mean learn as much as you can in order to ask the right questions from your health care providers and to actively participate in your treatment options and decision making.

- Don't listen to people who tell you all the horror stories they or their brother/mother/sister went through when they were diagnosed with cancer. Management of treatment side effects has improved tremendously over the years and everybody is different and reacts differently.

- Do what is best for you and listen to your body. Rest when you need to and do as much as you have the energy for.

- Don't hide your disease from others. Cancer is not contagious and having the disease is not your fault. However, don't be surprised if some people are very uncomfortable when they hear the news and distance themselves from you.

- Keep a positive attitude.

- You may have a melt down or two over the course of your diagnosis and treatment. This is perfectly normal. Don't beat yourself up over it and move on. It may even make you feel better by letting it all hang out.

- Last but not least, don't continually ask yourself "why me". It is just a waste of energy and there is no answer.

Roslyn Franken

Ottawa, Ontario.

Hodgkin's Disease Stage II

———■———

It was December 1994.

I was at a work conference in Florida and just returned to my hotel room after a magnificent beach party filled with music, dancing and laughter. I fell asleep high on life that night only to wake up at 3:00 am with a neck so swollen and painful that I could not lift my head up off the pillow. I tasted lobster for the first time that night and thought I was having an allergic reaction.

If only I had been so lucky.

I was rushed to the nearest doctor who put me on antibiotics hoping it was just a virus. It proved not to be a virus. I was then tested for mononucleosis. It wasn't a case of mononucleosis. The lump in my neck just kept getting bigger.

I was finally sent for an ultrasound, an experience I will never forget. The technician went about her business gliding the wand back and forth across my neck while looking at pictures on her screen. She then stopped suddenly and excused herself from the room without explanation. A male doctor took over and continued the procedure. I sensed something wasn't right. He muttered under his breath expressions like "Oh oh", "Mmmm", "Oh boy", "Oh dear".

I didn't say a word, but knew now something was wrong. He finished the procedure, told me that it looked like I might have "lymphoma", but only a biopsy can determine for sure and that I will be contacted to set up an appointment for the surgery. He then turned and walked out of the room.

I was 29 years old at the time and had no idea what the word lymphoma meant let alone biopsy. I wiped my neck of the ultrasound gel, got dressed, gathered my belongings and started heading out not knowing what to think or feel. I passed by the radiologist's office and saw him sitting at his desk. I couldn't help but poke my head in the door and ask him to define for me the words lymphoma and biopsy. His exact words were "Oh, lymphoma is cancer of the lymph nodes, but don't worry, you'll be fine". He barely looked up from his paperwork. He may have defined the word biopsy after that, but to be honest after the "C" word, I didn't really hear much of what he said. I walked out of his office numb.

As I drove home from the hospital, alone, trying to grasp and process the frightful news, a myriad of thoughts, emotions and questions washed over me like a tidal wave. My whole being was suddenly overcome with anxiety and an overwhelming fear of the unknown. "What's going to happen? What if I have cancer? Am I going to die? How am I going to tell my husband, parents, close friends, boss, and co-workers? How long will I have to wait till the biopsy?" These were just some of the questions pervading my mind. There were so many things to think about. It was hard to concentrate. I didn't sleep much that night.

My enlarged lymph node was removed during biopsy surgery. The pain following the surgery was more than I anticipated. As it turned out, the tumour was resting on the main artery to my brain, much deeper than the surgeon had realized. They had to cut through multiple layers of muscle just to reach it.

The biopsy results showed a clear case of Hodgkin's Disease Stage II, cancer of the lymph nodes. The treatment would involve chemotherapy to be administered once every three weeks for the next nine months. The oncologist explained what to expect from the treatments with all the miserable side effects -- including hair loss, nausea, fatigue, mouth sores, muscle spasms, back pain, and severe constipation, just to name a few -- all of which I experienced to varying degrees.

My life was forever changed after that moment in time. I will never forget what happened in those nine months and how it changed my life forever.

As I started my chemotherapy treatments, moment to moment survival became my new reality. I watched my hair fall out as it filled my pillow and went down the shower drain. I increased the fibre in my diet to combat the constipation, drank more water than you can imagine, and gave in to my body when it begged for rest. I took pills for nausea, pain control, constipation and to sleep better. My life revolved around looking after my physical well-being by "doing" all the "right" things.

I put on my wig and a smile each day and kept everything going as I'd always done before. I didn't know how else to be. I continued to work my full-time sales job, met all my quotas, and maintained my strong client relationships. From the surface, people wouldn't even know there was a problem. I just went about my life and work doing what needed to get done. I was so busy surviving day to day and trying to keep everything under control that I was completely oblivious to the emotional volcano that was bubbling up inside, until that one afternoon when it finally blew.

There I found myself one afternoon sitting on the floor, alone, in the middle of my living room enraged, crying uncontrollably, pleading unto God to help me understand and make sense of what was happening to me. I cried until my heart felt empty inside, and then eventually felt the waves of relief flow through me as my tears dried up and my heart slowly filled up again.

I was shocked by the intensity of emotions that exploded out from the depth of my soul. I felt confused. None of it made any sense.

After cooling down and reflecting on my unexpected outburst, a number of questions surfaced in my mind. "How could this be? Everything was going so well, right? Had I not been coping incredibly well with continuing to be a good wife, good daughter, good friend, good employee and good medical patient? Wasn't I always positive and brave? What was the problem? What else could I possibly expect from myself? Where was this overwhelming outpour of emotions coming from and how long had I been burying them inside? How were these feeding my cancer? How were these repressed emotions draining my inner spirit which I so badly needed in the fight for my life?" Asking myself these questions started a process of self-discovery and transformation that enabled me to step beyond my challenges and see myself, others and the world around me through a newer and wider lens of reality.

I wrote down my questions and just sat there with them. After a short while I started to write down whatever came to mind in response to the questions. I did not censor or judge what I wrote. I just kept the pen to the paper and kept on writing. It felt good to get it out. Later on in reading back what I wrote I came to understand myself on a whole new level. I was able to step beyond where I was in that moment to a whole new place of self-awareness and acceptance. It was a powerfully freeing experience that created a space for positive and meaningful change to take place.

I realized that I had been so busy trying to keep everything going as if nothing was wrong that I was not allowing myself to feel my true emotions. In trying to be strong and brave, take care of myself without asking others for help, and always wearing a smile, I was in fact unconsciously repressing my very real emotional pain and suffering. This was my turning point.

I wanted not only to understand my pain and suffering from a rational standpoint. I wanted to let go of whatever was preventing me from truly feeling the emotional pain.

For me this meant letting go of my need for control and independence. It meant accepting my humanness and vulnerabilities that this outburst was forcing me to face. It meant acknowledging and accepting my needs and desires for greater attention, care and support from my husband, family and friends. I hadn't realized till that point how much I needed and wanted to be loved and cared for without worrying about whether or not I was being a burden on the other person. Maybe others didn't realize how much I needed them because of my brave face. I knew it was up to me to reach out to them and let them know what I needed and wanted from them.

I could no longer worry about being a burden, and instead recognize that I am worthy and deserving of their time, love and attention. I was always there for my husband, family and friends in their times of need, so why shouldn't I have them there for me when I needed them most? When I did reach out, it was amazing how much care and support I received. It was also fascinating to see which friends stepped up to the plate and which ones didn't. I learned a lot not only about myself, but also about my friendships. I had some friends who made promises of how they would cook for me and help me out with other things, but not once did they live up to it.

Then there were others who came out of the woodwork, surprising me with meals, treats and coming over for visits. I also knew that I had to take more time to just "be" without feeling guilty if I didn't drink enough water that day, get enough sleep, or do everything exactly as I "should" be doing. I learned to let go of unproductive guilt and worry. I learned to stop trying to be so damn perfect and in control all the time.

In learning more about myself, I was able to see that my outburst was not a negative loss of control, but rather a positive release of repressed emotions. The process forced me to face my own humanness and vulnerabilities. It made me realize a need for change in how I was living with my cancer and processing the emotions around it. I could only imagine how these repressed emotions may have been contributing to the cancer and my healing process. I knew I would have to step beyond the surface and dig deep into the heart and core of my being to understand where I myself was coming from and what else needed to change.

The more I dug, asked myself questions, and explored each of the emotions, the more I was able to see the bigger picture and start to look for opportunities for positive and meaningful change. As my eyes opened, I was able to see, understand and appreciate myself and others through a clearer lens of reality. The cloud had lifted and light was now able to shine through once again. The process allowed me to break through my inaccurate views of myself and others and step beyond to greater happiness, depth and fulfillment. It allowed me to face my cancer with a truer sense of honesty, dignity and grace. By overcoming the "emotional" cancer that was eating me up inside, I was able to free my body, mind and soul to give the physical cancer a run for its money. I was able to focus on myself, but at the same time reach out to others when I needed help getting things done or simply even a shoulder to cry on.

As we've seen, what seemed like an insurmountable setback at first, turned out to be a launching pad into a whole awakening process that caused me to identify and challenge my beliefs, break negative patterns, take risks, and try on new behaviours. The cancer thus forced me to wake up, take notice and find my true self within. It was through the experience of my illness that I was able to accept and appreciate myself and my life in a fuller, truer and more meaningful way.

It was an empowering journey that enabled me to become a much stronger and more confident person walking on more solid ground, who could now overcome whatever obstacles life put on my path. I truly found my fighting spirit within.

It's now been more than ten years since my l;
in that time I have faced many more life sett
devastating divorce, job losses, a major car acc
of my mother to cancer in 2004 after an inspir;
21 year battle.

However, in that time, I have also had many triumphs to ᴄ
proud of. I went back to school and got my Masters degree in
Human Systems Intervention where I learned the theory and
practice of facilitating the processes of learning and change for
others. I then got my coaching certification wanting to work one
on one with people to help them in changing their lives, as I did
mine. I worked as a Life Coach helping others set and reach
their goals in their personal and professional life, but felt like an
imposter, frustrated with my own inability to reach my own goal
of wanting to shed the excess 40 pounds I had put on in the last
number of years.

I decided that in order to be as authentic as possible in helping
others reach their goals, I needed to be able to take care of my
own, as in "walk the talk", "practice what I preach". I'd already
had cancer, my mother had just passed away from cancer, so what
was I waiting for? That's when I put myself to task and finally
overcame my personal struggles with food and weight and decided
to counsel others to do the same. In September 2006, I released
my book, *The A List: 9 Guiding Principles for Healthy Eating and
Positive Living* and am now totally excited by what each new day
has to offer. If anyone would have told me even five years ago
that I would be a published author, counselor and motivational
speaker helping people eat better, feel better and live better, I
would have laughed out loud. You just never know where your
life experiences, seemingly good or bad at the time, are going to
take you. It is all what you make of them.

What I have come to know is that through continually
increasing my self-knowledge, challenging my beliefs, taking
risks and making changes where necessary, I continue to grow in
my ability to tackle life's adversities and step beyond them with

ɹ resilience. I've learned that life is seldom an easy ride. ᴡill always be challenges and obstacles to overcome, but it ɴow we rise to the occasion and in how we respond that will ɪke us or break us.

I believe that the process of stepping beyond our challenges is a continuous practice which can help get us through our difficulties, bouncing-back quickly, and prepared for whatever life brings next.

Surviving life setbacks in a meaningful way allows us to reframe suffering into challenge, failure into success and fear into strength. Through the lifelong practice of stepping beyond we can continue to find meaning and wisdom through our pains and struggles. The rewards can be tremendous. I now have more fulfilling relationships, a career that is rich in meaning and satisfaction, a healthy approach to problem solving, and am excited by all that life has to offer. This ongoing process enables me to continually strive to be fully human with an open mind, open ears and an open heart. It can do the same for you if you CHOOSE to allow it.

Roslyn Franken is author of The A List: 9 Guiding Principles for Healthy Eating and Positive Living. Roslyn offers private counseling and professional speaking services to those seeking healthy weight and positive lifestyle management for increased health and happiness. For more information, visit www.roselynfranken.com.

Jacquelin Holzman

Ottawa, Ontario

Ductal carcinoma in situ

————■————

The call from my doctor finally comes. "Jackie," he says, "I have bad news and I have good news. The bad news? You have breast cancer. The good news? It's the best kind: DCIS ductal carcinoma in situ. I've referred you to the Women's Breast Health Centre at The Ottawa Hospital."

In those few seconds, I'm on the road to becoming a cancer statistic!

Actually, the first step began during a regular mammogram a week earlier when the technician did extra filming. Always expecting the worst, I was suspicious. Knowing that my doctor had holidays scheduled, I asked his office to notify me by phone as soon as he got the results.

However, I can't say I was surprised by the diagnosis. I knew the risk factors, i.e. I was a woman, of "certain age" and, most important, my Mother had lost her fight with breast cancer in 1985.

But being intellectually aware of breast cancer and the resources available, hearing the words and my name in the same sentence, my stomach felt like it was in a vice, my tongue seemed to have doubled in size, my head started to spin and my breathing seemed to stop.

What should I do? How and what should I tell my family? And how will they react? Will they be as frightened as me?

Where is the instruction book? Who would give me the rules of the cancer world that I had just entered?

Since it was March, 1998, only four months since the end of my political career, having served for 15 years on Ottawa Council, the last six as Mayor, I believed that I still had a role to play in making a difference in people's lives.

Using my situation as a means of raising awareness for the need for early cancer detection, and encouraging women to get themselves checked, I put my face on breast cancer and decided to make a public announcement. It was not my style to hide my journey along the road as a cancer statistic. My husband and family agreed and promised their support.

In a month or so, the Ottawa Race Weekend would take place and, with the encouragement and assistance of the Ottawa Citizen, MDS Nordion and The Ottawa Hospital, my cancer was announced and a fund raising campaign was launched for the Women' Breast Health Centre as part of the Race Weekend. My daughter, Ellyn, accepted a challenge to run the 10 K and together we would raise money for the Centre.

If one wanted to raise awareness, where better than with a larger than life picture of my face on the front page of the Citizen above the fold!!!!

My personal journey along the road to my successful treatment and recovery was joined by hundreds of family, friends, professionals and organizations such as Breast Cancer Action. I learned that no one need travel it alone.

Well, as they say, the rest is history. Not only have my daughter and I raised over $200,000 for cancer care and research at The

Ottawa Hospital and the Ottawa Health Research Institute in the 10 years since the first Race Weekend, but hundreds of women brushed aside their fears and jammed the phone lines rushing to have their mammograms. Some even went as a group and had lunch afterwards!!

Each person will have a different experience when the word 'cancer' is linked with his or her name. Our reactions will not be the same. However, it should be reassuring for those who will become cancer statistics to know that more people are living after cancer treatment than dying.

Greater awareness on the importance of living a healthy lifestyle combined with the increased emphasis on developing new and quicker diagnostic techniques and more effective less invasive treatment offers hope for a future without cancer.

Cancer WILL be beaten!!!

Frank Hegyi

Ottawa, Ontario

Prostate Cancer

———————■■———————

In January 2004, Dr. Nancy Clevette, my Family Physician informed me that my PSA reading was 9.0 which was a bit high and suggested that I see a specialist. I was referred to a Urological Surgeon who scheduled a blood test for me and found that the PSA reading was now 9.5 It took another 6 months to have a biopsy which turned out to be a very painful experience, it lasted for about 15 minutes while the Doctor took samples through a tube inserted in the rectum. I was called in by the Urological Surgen's office for September 21st to get the news on the results of the biopsy. My daughter Jennifer came with me for the 4:30 pm appointment. Because of the time elapsed between the biopsy and my appointment was relatively long, I was pretty sure that the Doctor will tell me that I do not have prostate cancer. When it was time for me to go to the examining room, the nurse asked me if I wanted my daughter to be with me. I said no and told Jennifer that I will not be a minute to hear the good news. The nurse escorted me to the private office of the doctor. He asked me to sit down then looked at me in the eyes and said: "Mr. Hegyi, the biopsy results indicate that you definitely have prostate cancer". I almost fell off the chair. I had difficulty comprehending what the Doctor was telling me as I went into a deep shock. How could this happen to me, I don't smoke, I eat healthy food and I exercise. I am only 66 years old.

He explained further that since he is a surgeon, he would perform the radical prostatectomy. The surgery takes from 3-4 hours and recovery may take a few weeks. There is a chance that the nerves run along each side of the prostate gland down to the penis may get damaged, which would then result in impotency for life. The surgeon then suggested that I get independent advice from an oncologist about an alternative possible cure: radiation, after which I was to call him back concerning my decision.

When I went back to the waiting room, Jennifer saw on my face that the news was not good. I told her that I had prostate cancer and then she went into shock. When we got home, we told the news to my wife Rose who started to cry. I poured myself a stiff drink of rye, sat in my favourite chair pretending to watch the news on TV, but my thoughts were miles away. I was thinking of the discussion I had whith an old friend in 1973, Dr. Elizabeth Kübler Ross when we were discussing her new book "On Death and Dying" and especially the 5 stages terminal patients go through when they hear the "death sentence": denial, anger, bargaining, depression and acceptance. At that time I was a young scientist and the discussions were basically of academic interest, especially because my co-major for my M.Sc. degree was in bio-medical statistics. But now I found myself thinking about these stages with the feeling that I was looking into a mirror; for a moment the thought occurred that I may be terminally ill. Then, I looked at my 19 month old grandson (Ryan) and 2 months old granddaughter (Sara) who were in the room. I definitely wanted to live and decided that I will do whatever needed to be cured. I got strong support from my wife and daughter and Jennifer called her brother Mike and sister in law Penny and they also provided strong support by saying: "Dad, you are a survivor, you will beat this one, too. Besides, your two grandchildren here Nathan (17

years old) and Tassia (14 years old) expect you to be there
graduation." I told my son that they can count on that and
even be there when Ryan and Sara graduate.

Being a scientist by training, I decided to learn all I could
about this disease. So I carried out an extensive internet research
on prostate cancer, including what it is, how it spreads, what
treatments are available, what are the side effects and what are
the chances of survival. I found this to be very important so that I
could come to a decision on the treatment option that I would be
most comfortable with.

On October 5th I met Dr. Samant an oncologist at the Ontario
Regional Cancer Clinic (ORCC). Rose came with me to the clinic
and as I looked around, there were many patients who looked
rather ill, some without hair while others were in wheel chairs or
lying in bed with life supporting tubes as they were taken in for
radiation. Before seeing Dr. Samant, a Patient Designated Nurse
sat down with us and went over the Facts Sheet, we discussed the
Self Reporting Health History, and she gave us an overview of the
cancer services at ORCC. Then Dr. Samant and an intern came in
to talk to us about external beam radiation treatment, explained in
detail its side effects that included fatigue, skin reaction, bladder
irritation, bowel movement irregularity, possible impotence, and
rectal irritation. After that he did a DRE and confirmed that he
could not feel the tumour. I was then referred for another blood
test and scheduled to see Dr. Samant again on October 20th at noon
to confirm that I still want to take the external beam radiation
option. When I saw Dr. Samant on the 20th he had the results of
the PSA test at 9.2 and I said "great, my diet is working since the
PSA is coming down". He was quick to correct me that the .3
score drop does not mean anything, I still had the cancer. I told Dr.
Samant that I have definitely decided to take the radiation option.
He said that I will get good support, he will be there for me should
I run into complications.

Once I made a decision to take the external beam radiation
treatment, I also checked out how a change in diet could benefit

Cancer Survivors

' at their Will

weight

ated that a low-fat, high-fibre diet and regular prostate cancer cell growth by up to 30 percent. y attention to my food consumption and even ware package on internet called DietPower: ition Manager by DietPower Inc. Every day I recorded each food intake, including the amount, and drank lots of water.

My radiation treatment started January 27th, 2005. Rose came with me on this day which made it much easier because when you see other patients who are going for radiation after finishing chemo, the impact of cancer really hits home. A friend of mine who went through the radiation treatment suggested that I take with me my own dressing gown and slippers, psychologically it helps. I was glad that I took his advice, having my dressing gown was a lot more comfortable than those which the hospital provides. Then, I was escorted to one of four radiation rooms where there was a Primus Linear Accelerator equipment[1] to do the external beam radiation. I climbed up on the bench and lay face down, dressing gown pulled up, bare bottom exposed, and the radiation therapists were then positioning me to line up the tattoo marks on my behind for the radiation. This took about 3 minutes, then they told me not to move and placed the cold shell on me, strapped it down all around and said that they have to leave the room while the radiation takes place. The machine then moved around making different sounds as the radiation occurred, and 10-12 minutes later the therapists came back, un-strapped the shell, removed it, covered my behind with the dressing gown, and asked me to get down the same way as I got on the unit. I had to repeat this 5 times a week, and a total of 37 times. During this period, I also had to control my weight; it was not advisable to either gain or lose any weight in order to ensure that the radiation goes to the intended (marked) area. My computer software helped a lot in this regards.

---

[1] http://www.medical.siemens.com/webapp/wcs/stores/servlet/ProductDisplay?storeId
=10001&langId=-11&catalogId=-11&catTree=100001%2C12789%2C12757&level
=0&productId=17242

During the 10-12 minutes of radiation sessions when I was lying on the table motionless, I was reflecting about a lot of things that happened to me. The first thing that came into mind is that "will this work?" I spent some sessions in a state of despair and depression, thinking that how will I say goodbye to the family if they tell me that the radiation could not stop the spread of the cancer. I thought back to March 25th 1978 when I heard the news that the mother of my two children was in the hospital in Madison, Wisconsin, dying of cancer. We were divorced and I had custody of the children since they were 7 and 4. But, I made sure that the children would spend each summer with their mother. Now Michael was 16 and Jennifer was 13 years old. When I told them the news, Michael was crying and asked me to lend him the money so he can go to see his mother before she dies. Rose and I agreed that I should take them to Madison right away, and that I should be there with them when the end comes. On March 26th I took Michael and Jennifer by plane to Madison, we checked into a motel and stayed there during the whole time. Now I was fighting cancer, and was remembering the suffering that my ex-wife went through with the disease. She died 10 days after being admitted to hospital. On her final day just before the end came, she was heavily sedated with morphine, but the pain was still severe as she cried out "I am never going to leave this hospital alive". I was then allowed a few minutes of private time to say goodbye to her. She said "Look after our children for me". We then said goodbye, she knew the end was just a few minutes away and she was facing it bravely. I promised her that I will be there for the children and asked her to watch over them from heaven. Then, I took the children to the hospital chapel and we prayed that she be at peace and that God make her happy in heaven. We then went back to her room and she was finally at peace and I had to focus on comforting the children. These memories were so vivid, especially now that I was wondering if it is my turn now.

Most of the time when I went home after these sessions, Jennifer was there with the two grandchildren, Ryan and Sara.

Rose made supper for us and the grandchildren would sit on my lap and I was thinking how lucky I am to have the support of the family. Son Michael and daughter-in-law Penny were in touch by phone and e-mail every week, along with their children Nathan and Tassia. This was very important, especially as the side effects started to show up and get stronger each day. The treatment was usually between 4:30 and 5:30 pm, after that I go home, have dinner and would get into bed by 8 pm. After about 2 weeks of treatment, I was experiencing a lot of pain during bowel movement and the urination became frequent (at one and a half hour intervals, including during the night) and came with a burning feeling. By the end of each week, bowel movement would include passing quite a bit of blood, then the pain eased a little bit over the weekend.

On February 24th, 4 weeks into the treatment, I went for blood work and the results were given to me on March 9th. A ray of sunshine and hope suddenly came into my life when the nurse told me that the PSA came down to 6.5 However, I was cautioned that PSA reading can move up and down and it was too early to draw any conclusion. So, back in the "wait and see state" I went, getting increasingly fatigued and irritated as the side effects were having a field day with me. I had to be careful not to snap at people if they disagreed with me because my patience was wearing thinner as I was going through the second half of the treatment.

On March 17th I went for a blood test again then had the radiation. When I went home I was alone as I went to the bath room for a bowl movement that was particularly painful. After cleaning myself, I got up and noticed that I was bleeding heavily and continuously and this lasted for another half an hour.

My radiation treatment was completed on March 23rd but at that time I still not had the results of the PSA test. When I met with Dr. Samant that afternoon, he told me that the side effects will still be there for another 4-6 weeks, but if the radiation is successful, then the next PSA level should drop again. On March 31st got some good news that the PSA was down to 4.64 which meant that

I was responding well to treatment. Then I received further good news in May that the PSA level dropped to 2.72 and Dr. Samant was pleased about this development. I had another blood test on July 11th and received the results on July 20th the PSA level went further down to 1.0. It appears that I managed to beat cancer for a time being. Since my father, mother and grandfathers all died at 86 and now that the life expectancy is extended due to medical advances, diet and exercise, I consider that my expiry date will not come for at least another 20 years, which means that I can attend the University graduation of all the grandchildren. I was already fortunate to attend the High School graduation of my grandson, Nathan Hegyi in Waunakee, Wisconsin on June 5, 2005. What a proud time that was for me and I already promised Nathan to be there for him when he graduates from college. On August 18th I went back to Waunakee for 12 days to look after my 15 year old grand daughter Tassia while her parents took Nathan to Missoula, Montana to start his University education. He is enrolled to study photo journalism. I had a great time looking after Tassia, taking her to JV volleyball practices and games. I definitely have a lot to live for and very grateful to the staff at the Cancer clinic for the great job they have done. My message to men who are over 50, get an annual check-up and PSA test, cancer can be beaten if it is diagnosed early enough and if you lead a healthy life and exercise regularly.

I have taken the cancer treatment as a wake up call. In the summer I try to play golf once a week and when the weather is bad, I work out in a health club for an hour on the tread mill. I still watch my food intake and monitor it with the computer software. Interestingly, I even go to church on most Sundays. I see Dr. Samant every 6 months and the PSA reading in January 2008 was 0.56

On June 6th 2008 I attended my granddaughter's high school graduation and in June 2009 Nathan will be graduating from college. I am determined to attend Sara's college graduation (she is now 4 years old) right up to when she graduates with a PhD. degree.

Eating well, playing golf and controlling weight are all important ingredients of being a cancer survivor. Positive attitude and the determination to attend the graduation of my grand children have made my cancer journey much easier.

On May 4, 2008 (to celebrate my 70th birthday) my 5 year old grandson and I rode our bicycles in Tour Nortel 2008 for 12 K and raised $750 for the Children's Hospital of Eastern Ontario cancer research.

Cheryl Kardish-Levitan

Ottawa, Ontario

Breast Cancer. Invasive Ductal Carcinoma

———■———

I had been running for 21 years and had completed 20 marathons internationally and locally, as well as an equal number of half marathons. I love to run for fun, health, and to experience the runner's high.

I have been working out daily and even challenged myself to cycle from Ottawa to Kennebunkport, Maine, with my husband Brian in four days averaging 160 kilometres a day. I didn't realize that I would soon be facing the greatest challenge of my life.

I was feeling great. I was on the right track. But on June 30th, 2000 my course had changed directions and I was heading for a crash.

I had just come back from my run when I received a call from my physician telling me to sit down. The core biopsy I had two days earlier showed that my lump was a malignant tumour and that I had cancer.

I thought this was a mistake, because the mammogram and ultrasound that I had the week before were just routine.

The core biopsy was just to verify that whatever I had was a cyst and it was benign, like 90% of them. Anyway, the mammogram that I had 6 months earlier had been clear. I was so sure that it was just a simple procedure that I told my husband not to bother coming with me because there was nothing to worry about.

The doctor kept on talking to me, but nothing he said registered except that I had CANCER. I was in shock, paralyzed, as if I were having an out of body experience.

All I could think about was I MAY DIE! The doctor apologized for telling me on the Friday before the long weekend because he knew that my three children were leaving for a month at sleep-away camp.

I kept on thinking: I'm too healthy, I never smoked, I don't drink, I lead a very healthy lifestyle, and there was no immediate family history of cancer.

Two of my children were with me at the time, and they are very perceptive and could tell something was wrong. I dropped them off at the video store and called Brian to tell him the devastating news.

When I arrived home I ran upstairs to my bedroom and we just hugged each other and cried.

We realized we had to first tell our children, Elana 15, Tyler 13, and Ian, 9, each separately before they left for camp. We have a very large extended family-well over 100 members- and we didn't want them to hear the news from anyone else.

This was one of the most difficult and emotional moments for me because I had to put on a very brave face. I told them I had a small tumour, but that I had the best doctors. I promised them that I would be okay. I reassured them that I would beat this, like my aunt did 26 years ago when she had a radical mastectomy and chemo and just celebrated her 50th wedding anniversary.

My family knew I was a fighter and I knew that this was going to be the greatest challenge I would ever have to face. This was not going to be like any marathon or triathlon that I ever trained for. I didn't realize at the time that all of my years of training for long endurance runs, discipline, meditating on those two four-hour runs would be my new training and coping skills to help me prepare for the Run of My Life!

The next morning we called my doctor at home to have him explain exactly what kind of cancer I had. He told us that I had Invasive Ductal Carcinoma, and that the cancer had spread outside the ducts. The tumour was close to two centimetres. The word invasive is very scary when you are not educated or informed about cancer, especially when there are more than 150 different kinds of tumours.

On Sunday we took our children to the camp buses and I hugged, and kissed them goodbye. What was going through my mind was, 'Will I be around in the next few years to see them grow up and see them get married? Not knowing what you are fighting is fearful.

When you find out that you have a life-threatening disease you immediately get a reality check. Nothing is more important than understanding your role and taking control of your own health. In training for a marathon no one can log those miles for you; you alone have to train and put in those long distance runs.

I knew that no matter how many people wanted to help me - and I had an amazing support network - I alone had to initiate my own healing journey.

I've been very fortunate to have one of the foremost breast surgeons as my long-time friend. When I phoned him and told him of my diagnosis, he met with me immediately and eased my fears. He also presented the various options open to me and showed me the tumor so I could feel it for the first time. I had to decide if I wanted a mastectomy or a lumpectomy with radiation and possible chemotherapy and tamoxifin, as adjuvant therapies, if required. I read all of the medical information available.

I had a date set for my surgery, five weeks away, on August 2nd. Of course I wanted the treatment that was going to give me the best chance for survival. I was surprised to learn that both choices gave the same percentages.

After several weeks of reading and researching everything I could get my hands on, I opted for a lumpectomy with the additional removal of lymph nodes under my arm which meant I would definitely need radiation therapy and possibly chemotherapy.

I decided that from that moment on I was going to be in control of how I would respond to the ways in which cancer was going to change my life forever.

When I decided to run my very first marathon there was a steep learning curve characterized by the usual mistakes, setbacks, frustrations, and hard won rewards of any worthwhile experience. That was the exact same path that my journey with cancer would follow.

I decided to work until the day before my surgery. As soon as the news spread about my diagnosis, the phone did not stop ringing. Emotionally drained, we decided to take a much-needed vacation to Cancun.

It was the best decision we made, and turned out to be the most wonderful vacation.

I put my fear of cancer in a compartment and appreciated and cherished every moment we spent together. I came back 10 days before my surgery in a positive frame of mind.

The outpouring of emotional support from friends, family and business colleagues were overwhelming and humbling. The day before my operation I opened up a spirit-boosting e-mail from one of my real estate clients:

Hi Cheryl,

I just learned that you will be having some surgery in the near future. This is one of those times when you need to reflect on your marathon training. Running a marathon is the ordinary person doing the extraordinary.

Beating breast cancer is all about your mental toughness combined with the support of family, friends and quality of medical care... Cheering you to the finish line in your race against breast cancer will be the loud voices of all of the team at the Running Room.

John Stanton,

John Stanton is the CEO of The Running Rooms across Canada and is a major sponsor for the Run for the Cure and donates $10.00 of every piece of clothing that has the pink ribbon on it to breast cancer. Last year they contributed $100,000. I am proud of what he does for this cause and was able to participate in this past year's Run for the Cure and raise over $2,000 myself.

My surgery was very successful; my tumour was only 1.3 centimetres and I had eight lymph nodes removed.

I had gotten through the first half of the marathon-my tumor was removed and now I had to prepare for the finish, getting through the radiation treatments and dealing with the results of my pathology report.

Not knowing how bad the prognosis was, the eight days following my surgery were difficult. I decided I would face it head on. I tried on wigs, and did a lot of soul searching, visualization and positive self-talk. I took mega-doses of vitamins, minerals and immune-building teas like essiac. I said a prayer every morning and night. I made a list of superstar affirmations that I repeated daily on my runs, at night and in my car.

My results were remarkably good. I had stage 1 cancer and a very rare tumour that only two per cent of women yearly are diagnosed with. It was a tubular. I had no cancer in any of my lymph nodes. My prognosis was fantastic. I had a 10% chance that the cancer could return. Surgeons and oncologists always deal in percentages; chemo and tamoxifen for me would reduce that 10% to 7%.

Overcome with gratitude and relief, I felt blessed with a second chance at life. The right decision for me, which I had thought about for weeks, was radiation therapy and my medical team supported it.

I started my radiation treatments in late September and went everyday except on weekends for six weeks.

The first time I went to get marked was very emotional. You feel so vulnerable as they mark up your breast and surrounding area with magic marker and get your co-ordinates for the simulator radiation room.

Thank goodness they have patience and a sense of humour. My marks totally smeared after my first run and I had to go back to get re-marked. After I started, they figured they should put tape on top of my marks since they hadn't experienced any patients who continued running throughout their therapy.

I was totally honest and open about what was happening to me emotionally, mentally, and physically. I would show my scars and marks to anyone who wanted to see them. My surgeon performed not just a life saving operation in my mind but also did a work of art.

Support is a crucial part of your healing and recovery. My husband was amazing in the constant love, caring, nurturing and support he gave to me. My children picked up the slack and continued to shower me with hugs and kisses. Rabbi Bulka was there for me from the moment he heard of my diagnosis. I can't praise enough or express my gratitude to Dr.Mark Hardy, my surgeon, Dr.Norman Barwin my Physician, Dr Roanne Segal, my medical oncologist, Dr. Paul Genest, my radiation oncologist, Dr.Mary Ann Mucha and the rest of the medical support team.

We are very fortunate to have one of the best cancer clinics in the country.

My friends and family were my Rock of Gibraltar. My best pal, my dog Zoe, a King Charles Cavalier spaniel, was my constant companion throughout my ordeal.

It's sort of like hitting the wall at mile 21 of a marathon. When you are just so tired and all of your muscles are aching, you just want to stop and give up- but you know that the pain is worth it to reach your goal.

The strategy that worked for me was to continue to try to maintain my level of fitness by running, walking, and weight training for my arm as much as I could.

Not only the hardest challenge I've ever faced, cancer has been the best and most rewarding marathon I've ever finished. I have come through this journey with a new commitment to life and as a much stronger person.

I must reflect that since my first Run For The Cure I have raised over $90,000 for breast cancer research and hope to reach my initial goal of $100,000 for this years run. Raising money for breast cancer has become my new passion since surviving breast cancer and being on the breast cancer Dragon Boat Team called Busting Out. I feel it is my duty to give back and in my own small way make a difference to help find a cure for this insidious disease.

I am now back to running full marathons and hope to complete my #26th Marathon at the end of this month in Ottawa's National Capital Marathon. I just came back from doing an extreme hiking trip for one month in New Zealand and skydived from 13,000 feet. I am living each day to the fullest and am grateful for everyday.

Barry Bokhaut

Ottawa, Ontario.

Esophageal cancer

———■———

W hen I received the terrifying news that I had esophageal cancer in the year 2000, I did as much research as possible to find out more about my illness. What I discovered was terrifying; the estimates from the Cancer Society statistics gave me a less than a 5 % chance of survival. Other sources were less optimistic, and indicated that the mortality equalled the incidence. That's a nice way of saying that there were no survivors for more than five years.

A key to surviving cancer is to have a positive attitude. That was pretty difficult given the reality of my disease. Rather than dwell on doom and gloom, I decided to seek success stories. I felt that if I could find one or two survivors with my type of cancer, then I could be hopeful that I would have a chance of making it.

There was only one person I knew who had oesophageal cancer, the Right Honourable Herb Grey, deputy prime minister of Canada. I didn't think it was likely that he would be available to chat if I called him to talk about our common illness. My wife heard about Peer Support, a service of the Canadian Cancer Society, and she called to find out if there was a cancer survivor that I could speak with. A few days later I received a call from George, in his seventies, a 12 year oesophageal cancer survivor.

Our conversation was not lengthy, George was up at his cottage chopping wood, and he wanted to finish before it got dark. That's all I really needed to hear. There was a long term survivor who was back to a normal lifestyle. George provided me with the hope that I needed, and allowed me to dream that I too would survive, despite the overwhelming odds.

My cancer journey was gruelling; filled with months of radiation and chemotherapy sessions after very invasive surgery that removed most of my oesophagus, formed part of my stomach into an oesophagus, and moved what was left of my stomach up into my chest. The stress of the treatment was likely a factor in the heart attack that I suffered. But I was buoyed by the knowledge that there were survivors of my disease, and I was determined that I was going to be one.

Once on the road to recovery, I realized just how important it was for me to have spoken to a survivor of my illness. I decided that it was time to pay back the generosity I had received from my peer support volunteer, and I signed up to provide support to others who were suffering from esophageal cancer. I also made a side deal with my "maker". I pledged that if He allowed me to survive, I would make myself available to speak to anyone who could benefit from my experience. Doing so would somehow provide me with some consolation for having had to go through this terrible journey. And it would provide an answer to the question " Why me?" and more importantly, "why did I survive when so many other have not".

I found it easy speaking to the people had asked for my help. I had become knowledgeable and a excellent resource simply because I had gone through the same experience they were going through, or were about to face. I provided them with the facts that they needed to know. We discussed the difficult, life and death decisions they had to make. We did this calmly and rationally.

I related well to the people I was counselling because of our shared experience, I outwardly showed little compassion or sympathy for their situation, even though I was deeply moved by their predicament. They weren't looking for a shoulder to cry on. They had friends or relatives who were available to listen and feel sorry for them, to console them. Our conversations focused on providing details of what their treatment was going to involve, based on what I had experienced. We spoke of the heart wrenching decisions that would have to be made about the choices in treatment. Because esophageal cancer is so aggressive, we spoke about the need to make these difficult decisions quickly, without having the benefit of lengthy consultations, numerous medical opinions or the luxury of sitting back and thinking about what to do.

Those who I have counselled have thanked me for speaking with them openly, for allowing them to ask personal questions about my experience. I caution them that I am not a doctor, and that I can not provide any medical advice. I stress that it is their doctors' advice and guidance that they must follow, as their doctor is the expert. This is understood, yet they felt that I could answer some questions better than by their doctor because I had personally gone through the experience. I was able to discuss details of their treatments and speak about the emotional and personal aspects of their cancer, giving them the time that their doctor could not be expected to give them. I perhaps most importantly, I was able to give them confidence, the same confidence that I had received in speaking to my peer support volunteer.

I was often surprised to hear that the person I was counselling felt that I was upbeat and positive, even though we had spoken about very grim scenarios without undue optimism. I make it a point to speak to these people openly, honestly and with brutal frankness. I always preface our discussions with the proviso that if our discussion becomes too intense or becomes too disturbing, that we can drop the topic and move on to something else with no explanations needed. In virtually every instance, my frankness in speaking about the issues has been appreciated and encouraged; they want to hear about and discuss what they will be facing without a sugar coating, and without false hopes or unwarranted encouragement.

I am motivated to provide peer support because I know that it helps others cope. The realization of how much peer support helps shocked me when I received a call from the wife of a cancer patient I had supported a while back. She called because her husband had passed away, and he wanted me to know that he had lost his battle. When I had asked about funeral arrangements, she said that they had not been considered yet; he had just passed away. Although I was neither family nor a friend, I was one of the first people that was called to share the sad news. I had truly made a difference in the lives of this couple.

Peer support has helped me deal directly with my ongoing battle with cancer. Although it is seven years since diagnosis, I still have issues with nutrition and stamina. I frequently have episodes where I suddenly experience complete exhaustion and weakness, dizziness and profuse sweating. I have consulted a number of medical specialists who could not provide a reason for this condition, and therefore could not recommend a treatment. Special diets, vitamin injections, nutritional supplements were all tried with very little success.

I was able to find the reason for my condition when I was discussing the condition of a peer support client I was counselling. I wasn't familiar with the terms he was using, so I went online to get information. As I was poking around, I came across a condition called late dumping syndrome. The symptoms were those that I was experiencing, and are found in those who have had their digestive systems compromised because of disease or surgery. I would not have been able to find a diagnosis of my problem if I had not had the opportunity to provide support to someone else.

I shed a tear when I learn of the outcome of my peer's condition; a tear of joy when they survive, even if it is for a little while, and a tear of sadness when I learn that they have succumbed. Providing peer support is emotional, and draining. Yet it is a wonderfully uplifting experience. It makes me realize how fortunate I am to be a survivor. My life has been changed because of cancer, and I have lost the ability to enjoy life as fully as I hoped I would be able to. Being a peer support volunteer, I can ignore what I have lost, and appreciate the wonderful life that I am able to live.

The bond that develops between those who have traveled the harrowing road of cancer is unbelievably strong. I mentioned that I didn't think that the Deputy Prime Minister of Canada would be concerned about my illness. I had the opportunity to speak to Mr. Grey a few years after my diagnosis, and I mentioned that I had contemplated asking him to visit me, but thought it was an unreasonable request. He looked me straight in the eye and said "you should have called, I would have come". Five years after diagnosis, I had a party to celebrate my survival, and the fact that I was considered cured of cancer. I invited Mr. Grey. Although he didn't know me, our cancer connection was strong, and he and his wife attended our joy of being survivors.

Barbara

Breast Cancer. Ductile carcinoma.

———————■———————

I was diagnosed with breast cancer almost nine years ago, November 1999. My GP found a lump in my left breast during my annual examination that had not been there before, so as a precaution she suggested that I have an ultrasound. As it turned out a mammogram was required and a biopsy, and both tests confirmed that yes, I had breast cancer. So my journey down the dark road of dealing with breast cancer began. When my surgeon told me I had to have my total breast removed because of the type of cancer I had, ductile carcinoma in situ, my first reaction was one of disbelief. My comment to my doctor was, "My husband doesn't want me whole, who is going to want me now with only one breast?" His response, in a polite version, was that my husband wasn't worth the ground he stood on and that a real man would love me for me, not my parts or in this case, missing part. After 23 years of marriage, I had been turned in for a much younger model the month before receiving this news, I was in shock. Now what – how was I going to tell my daughters this latest tidbit? We were already struggling with the separation and all felt totally abandoned. But as I have found over the last few years, you just get on with it. I think I came to terms with all of this by telling myself that I have cancer, breast cancer, I can either become a victim or I can deal with this the best way I can. While there was lots of tears, choking tears in the shower so my girls wouldn't hear me – I kept telling myself that I had to be strong for the three of us. To be honest, there was just so much to deal with, I think life became a blur for the next few months. Our first Christmas without the presence of husband and father was going to be difficult enough, let alone having my mastectomy booked for January 4th. My surgeon was wonderful, he gave lots of advice and support, he checked and verified that the route recommended was the only route to go by testing and retesting. He called my girls and reassured them and inquired how they were doing both before and after my surgery. But we did get through it with the help of family and friends; in particular my brothers. My mother's reaction was unsettling, her comment was, "oh dear don't let them take your breast away!" My mother has generally dealt with life's spin balls by pretending they aren't as bad as they actually are or dismissing them altogether. While my husband thought this was my attempt to get him back, he soon learned it was not and we, my daughters and I, soon learned he was to be no help to any of us. My family and girlfriends became my support team and a long time family friend stepped up to the plate once he found out that my husband had moved on. This friend became my strength right along with my family and friends. He made me feel like a million bucks, and helped me regain my self confidence and pride. He taught me that it was the person I was inside that counted, not the outside physical appearance which I now looked at in horror. Like everything else in life, time is a great healer and the absence of my left breast became less of a shock. My newly acquired prosthesis grew to be my new bud and I actually started to feel that I looked "normal" again. Breast cancer was just one of several issues I had to deal with at the time, but we got through it. Adjusting to the changes in my person, my home, my life got easier over time. The selling of our family home, uprooting my daughters from a single home to a small townhouse miles away from their friends was to be a turn in the road and my journey in life.

The closing of the door in Manotick and opening the door in our new neighbourhood in Stittsville was to be a new beginning – new friends, new neighbours, new adventures, a new me. Being the new females on the block made us the interest of some of the male neighbours. For all those things my husband used to do – repair this, fix that – there was no end of available help. In time I could see, as could my friends, a growing confidence in myself and in my abilities – I was a survivor in more ways than one.

The time had come for me to decide on reconstruction or not. Being single there was no question in my mind what I was going to do. Breast Cancer Action was a wealth of information and support. I did a lot of research through books and the internet as I wanted to have the most natural looking and feeling breast that I could. I called several people that I heard of through word of mouth and found that I was able to ask total strangers about their experience – pros and cons. I even met with Ottawa's former mayor, Jacquelin Holzman and had a show and tell session with her. She and her husband were very frank about her/their experience. In the end I chose what happened to be an invasive solution but one that was using only natural, not artificial input. And once again, I saw a change for the better and I felt like a new woman – I even acquired a nipple tattoo to complete the new look! My surgeon did a wonderful job but in hind site, I don't think that I would have chosen this procedure if I knew what I know now – my stomach will never see flat days again!

At a support group for breast cancer patients run by the Civic Hospital I discovered "Busting Out," a group of breast cancer survivors who paddled dragon boats. Never being what one would refer to as being athletically inclined, I thought I can do this, I want to do this. The first introduction to these crazy ladies was a hike in the Gatineau coupled with a pot luck lunch. These women shared stories of how some of them dealt with Chemo hair, prosthesis mishaps, family, work, and in general, their changed life, and this made me want to sign up then and there. Little did I know what joining this group of women was going to do for me and that my life was about to change in ways I never dreamed of. Over the past 9 years with these ladies I have become part of a top notch team of survivors, breast cancer survivors. The coaches recognized our desire to succeed and to be more than an advertisement for life after breast cancer and trained us to be our individual best. And the best it was to be because in 2005 we won a gold medal in Vancouver at the first international breast cancer survivor dragon boat competition. Then in September 2007, we travelled to Australia as a team to compete in the second international breast cancer survivor competition. No gold medals this time, but lots of good memories. By joining this team of positive thinking and active women, I have made many friends for life. Women that I am proud to say are my friends, my team mates, my support, my sisters. We laugh, we cry, we sympathize, we encourage one another to be our best. No expectations, you is who you is!

While having cancer might be labelled by some as a death warrant, for me it was a blessing in disguise. I have had reconstructive surgery, I am the proud owner of a new perky breast, I live a normal life and I don't obsess about cancer. My daughters have grown up to be lovely women – my pride and joy and my greatest accomplishment so far. While I may not have found my new life partner, I now know what I am worth and exactly what I have to offer that special somebody. I would have never won a gold medal, I would have never travelled to Australia as part of a team to compete internationally, and I would not have had the opportunity to meet these wonderful women had I not had breast cancer.

Do I think about recurrence – of course I do and more so with time mainly because more and more members of my dragon boat team are going through not only one recurrence but sometimes two and three. Several of my team mates get my total admiration – they accept what has been thrown at them in their journey through life and have tackled it with both barrels loaded. While they may be screaming on the inside, they put forth a strong and determined appearance on the outside and they are still here paddling their hearts out. I know that I am in the cancer game and there is no easy way out. If the cancer returns, I'll deal with it the best I can knowing that I have a whole new team, my Busting Out buddies to help me through.

Life has handed me some lemons but I happen to prefer lemonade!

Bob Carty

Ottawa, Ontario

Colon cancer

———————◼◼———————

It was a Thursday morning, and I had no premonition.

In fact, several days earlier I had called the doctor who did my colonoscopy. He had taken several samples of a particular polyp and I was anxious to know what the biopsies had found.

"Do you have any results?" I asked his nurse. Yes, she replied, the results had come in and the doctor would be in touch. Well, he didn't call. Not that day or the next. So, figuring that bad news travels fast in health matters, I took this as good news. The biopsies were probably negative – no cancer.

So on Thursday morning, January 4, 2007, I was pretty sure that all was well. Then the call came. "I'm sorry but I have some bad news," the doctor said directly. "Of the samples we took several were quite normal. But two turned out abnormal."

"What does that mean, 'abnormal'," I asked. "Well, they're not healthy cells. In fact, they're cancerous," he said. Further imaging tests would need to be done, he noted. But there was no doubt. You have cancer.

I put down the phone after the call. I sat at my desk. Not really feeling or thinking anything. But my body was surely reacting: heart pumping, breathing a bit strained, a cold sweat on my skin. Slowly some focus came back - what does this mean? The possibility of death? And short of that, the end of my career at CBC radio? Perhaps the fading of all the expectations I had only begun to form about enjoying this stage of life?

A deep breath. Keep moving.

At this point the hardest part was telling others. First my family. My spouse and son were very supportive, taking it well I thought. Though I did notice the house seemed to become quieter, as if they were bowled over by what this means for us as family, and by what I will need of them.

More deep breaths. Keep moving. There were doctors to see, people who had to be informed. And a list of legal paperwork I had always put off – power of attorney, last will and testament, making sure all my documents were in order. And then there were all the simple tasks in life - family shopping, giving a ride downtown for my son, rehearsing music for the local church. I can do this, I told myself. Though now there was a dark shadow hanging over everything.

About four days after getting the news I took a leave from the CBC and told my colleagues at work. They are more than work-mates – friends. They seemed effusive with condolences and expressions of care. But you quickly appreciate that there are only so many things to say at times like these. It was hard for me to keep repeating the news, person after person, day after day. At the same time I know it was hard for others to take it in. I'm sure they all must have wondered how best to respond.

Some reactions were troubling. Upon hearing the news one friend immediately morphed into the role of 'counsellor': "This is an experience that for some reason you are meant to take and from which you will gain new gifts. It's a wonderful journey," she said. Excuse me? If it's a journey, let *me* discover it; but at that moment I wasn't seeing cancer as good news. And I didn't need that kind of "encouragement."

One of my relatives thought the best way to respond was with matter-of-fact bravado: "Oh, you'll probably go under the knife, but, who knows, you might not need a bag (a colostomy) for the rest of your life."

I found that I most appreciated those people who just listened, carefully and with sympathy.

The worst was telling my mom. She's 84, in very good health and her seven adult children are free from life-threatening diseases. Now I have to deliver this news, thinking, as I was making the phone call, about how parents are supposed to die before their children. I can't forget the way she sighed and said "Oh, Bob."

In retrospect I was in a purple funk for about five days. No energy. Fairly depressed for someone who usually doesn't get down. I did some research on the Internet, especially looking at survival rates (very good for stage one, over 90% - not so good for stage four – under 8%). Ouch. What stage do I have? It would be several more weeks before finding out. This was beginning of one of the hardest parts of dealing with cancer – **the waiting**.

I don't know why this happened, but on the fifth day, I had a bit of a breakthrough. I went to a coffee shop and got a green tea to go. I went out to the waterfall at Mooney's Bay on the Rideau River here in Ottawa. And I just sat there in the car, sipping tea. It was a very cold January day, but sunny. I did some deep breathing.

And in that space I found a certain kind of *centeredness*. I recognized it as something I had felt before in periods of spiritual reflection and meditation – and maybe that's one reason I was able to pull it out of the recesses of my mind and heart. It was a simple sense of acceptance and gratitude - that even if this is the end of my life, it has been a good life. Despite all the failures and things undone, I've run a pretty good race. I could live with that – I guess I could die with that.

In the following days I tried to answer that difficult and nagging question that all cancer patients face – *why me*? There was no family history of this kind of cancer. But, as an investigative journalist, I was starkly aware of how much we have allowed industry to pollute our water and air and food with carcinogens. And I had also chosen to live parts of my life in Central America, one of the most pesticide-soaked regions of the world. And then there's diet … and life-style … and bad luck … and, who knows?

I was 57-years old and the only visits I had ever made to hospitals were to see friends or relatives, or to sing Christmas carols to the patients. And I had been feeling pretty good. The previous August, my son, Michael, and I did a four-day camping trip on the French River. It was strenuous but invigorating. At work I felt almost at the top of my game – doing quality work, respected by colleagues, taking on some challenging investigations and documentaries, even doing some teaching.

Then, in September, I noticed a little blood in my bowel movements. And I was feeling tired, unable to do much exercise. My mind felt unfocussed at work. I called my family doctor. It was probably the best medical decision I've ever made. At the family health clinic they immediately concluded I needed a colonoscopy. A requisition would go in right away.

But the clinic had trouble getting a response from the gastroenterologist they usually consulted. When he finally responded it was to say that he could only do the colonoscopy in six months due to his waiting list. When my doctor's office relayed this information, I was prepared. I had done my homework. Passing blood is serious, a possible indication of a tumour. And I had conducted enough interviews within the health care system to feel confident in pushing where push is needed. I insisted that they hunt around for another doctor to do the procedure. Waiting half a year was not an option. That was perhaps my second best decision.

Sure enough, in a few days they found a doctor who had just returned to Ottawa from Toronto - and he hardly had a waiting list at all. I would be in for the colonostomy within three weeks from that point.

On November 22, during my first colonoscopy at the Ottawa Hospital, the GI doctor removed five polyps. I watched it all on TV. It was not nearly as difficult as I imagined – a bit uncomfortable at moments (it's the air they pump in), but manageable. In fact, the worst part was taking the purging chemicals the previous day to clean out your entire system.

The GI doctor was quite happy with the five polyps he had snipped out. But he was concerned about a sixth polyp – or maybe it was not a polyp at all, but something else. It looked different. He took some photographs and some samples for analysis.

About a week later, the GI doctor called to say all samples sent to pathology came back "normal." But he still didn't like the look of that sixth growth. He wanted to do another colonoscopy to take more samples.

Well, due to the usual wait (and, on my part, getting a winter flu) it took until December 21 to be scheduled. Multiple samples were taken from the growth. The GI doctor said he wanted me to have a CT scan immediately. But of course there were no CT scans being done over Christmas.

Which brings us to the morning of January 4, 2007, and the "you have cancer" call. The doctor apologized for giving such bad news but he hoped we had caught it in time.

A CT scan was now imperative. Which was a perfect moment for a bit of irony: Ottawa's CT scan programme was undergoing "corporatization" – a centralization of systems to make the booking of scans more *efficient*. This efficiency measure, however, meant another delay in getting my scan.

Again, I made a few insistent phone calls. And the CT scan did happen on January 15th, 2007. Immediately afterwards, a surgeon told us he could see what looked like a two-inch (5 cm) tumour about 4 inches (10 cm) into my rectum. He would consult with other doctors.

Things then started to move quickly – and with much more technical detail. I had an MRI. Then separate consultations with a surgeon, a radiation oncologist and a chemo specialist. They said the tumour looked small but it may have affected two lymph nodes nearby which seemed enlarged. At that point they were calling it a Stage III rectal cancer (though final staging is only confirmed after surgery and pathology work).

Now, Stage III is certainly better than Stage IV (metastasis to other body organs), but it's not as good as Stage II. And you can't help but *Google* up the survival rates. And worry.

So I decided to go to the meetings of the local support group of the national colorectal cancer association. These are gatherings of colon cancer survivors and current patients undergoing treatment – everything from Stage I to Stage IV. Courageous people. And people willing to discuss the most difficult details of their health and how they have been struggling with various kinds of treatments. Here, there were no awkward reactions to your predicament. And there was a wealth of knowledge and experience - which doctors in the city are the best, how do you get a referral, which drugs should I fight for …

In my own case, before serious treatment, I needed a bit more biopsy work and a bone scan, plus the marking of my tumour with an ink stain so it could be found upon later surgery.

Then, in the first week of March, I finally got started. A five-and-a-half week programme of chemo and radiation at the same time. I was fortunate that my health plan covered the cost of oral chemo (about $1,400 for the 5 ½ weeks), which meant I could escape the uncomfortable standard treatment of a Picc line (a peripherally inserted central catheter – basically a tube from your left upper arm into the top of your heart) and chemo pump on a leash). At the same time I got radiation every working day with weekends off. With my kind of cancer, surgery would be after the chemo and radiation.

As a new student of cancer therapy I learned that the combination of radiation with chemo drugs is apparently done for two reasons – the chemo weakens cancer cells in the radiated area so the radiation is more effective, and it also kills other cancer cells traveling around the body. As someone who observes human behaviour for a living, I was overwhelmed by the number of people who came forward to offer help – cooking meals, providing rides, lending books and music. The love was over-flowing.

But the side-effects were brutal. There was nausea – you have to force food down if you can manage it. But most of all there was fatigue – a deep weakness really. They tell you that you will feel tired, but that does not prepare you for the totally debilitating impact of the treatments. I walked like an old man, lost my breath after one flight of stairs, sometimes got dizzy and often lost my concentration (though it's only fair to admit I already had some of these characteristics). But in other ways I couldn't complain – I only had a few mouth sores, I kept my hair (still greying though) and my finger tips, though a bit blistered, were still up for some banjo and guitar playing. Curiously, it was not over when the 5 ½ weeks of treatment stopped – the fatigue and side-effects actually got worse for another two weeks.

Then, finally, I started to feel better. Able to take a good long walk, sit in the sun, even do some exercises. I was waiting for a surgery date.

I had been assigned a surgeon by the cancer system. But he would not do this kind of rectal surgery laparoscopically. And as a journalist I had become a fan of minimally invasive surgery. It just made sense – less recovery time, sometimes less recurrence of the disease. So I talked to my family doctor and insisted on a referral – two in fact. In the end I interviewed three surgeons. And I chose the one with the most experience in a laparoscopic approach. He also had the best interpersonal skills.

The surgery was on June 4th. Three little incisions, some air pumped in to inflate the abdomen area, and then the section of the rectum where the tumour was located was taken out (about 8cm of rectum and colon in all). And then the piping was reconnected with about 120 titanium staples.

I emerged from surgery with just three little holes in an aging body and with a new appreciation for drugs derived from poppies or their chemical relatives. But I felt better, hour by hour.

Originally, they thought the surgery went well. When they went in they couldn't even find the tumour – the radiation had zapped it into non-existence. And the lymph nodes they took out for testing all came back negative for cancer. I was out of hospital in three days. A poster boy for rectal cancer and laparoscopic surgery.

I took in a neighbourhood picnic on day six. Started walking in the morning of day seven. But then, around day nine, the pain began. Slowly at first. Pain right at my tail bone. But my surgeon was now on holiday with his family. And I was only on Tylenol 3s (and not enough of them at that) and so spent a lot of days curled up on the couch with alternating applications of heating pads or bags of frozen peas wrapped in a towel. It went on for almost two weeks. About the worst experience of my life. I now realize I was just sucking up the pain like guys are supposed to do - insisting to myself that this was just a natural process of healing. Refusing to go to the emergency ward. The worst decision I made.

When my surgeon returned to work and heard about my pain he immediately had me admitted to hospital. That was July 4th. They ordered a CT scan and sure enough, there was a problem. On the circle of staples that reconnected the colon and rectum after the tumour was removed, at least one of the staples had failed. This was always a possibility with colon surgery (20-25%) and surgeons said it was often the result of the radiation treatment that weakened the flesh and made it unable to hold the staples. It may also have simply been a mechanical failure of a staple.

The result was a leak of gas and liquid from the bowel into the pelvic cavity just in front of the tail bone. In effect it created an abscess. There was a two-inch (5 cm) diameter cavity sitting behind the rectum and on top of a bundle of nerve endings. The result was pain equivalent to having an abscessed tooth - though obviously at the other end of things. And the potential for a disastrous infection.

I was immediately put on antibiotics and taken off any food or liquid for eight days (they did give me an intravenous saline solution). They were worried that the leaked waste matter could cause an infection and then septic shock, possibly death. That didn't happen - perhaps my one share of good luck. And besides, the diet was a guaranteed weight reduction plan.

The surgeon then took me back to the OR on July 9th to do a colostomy (the reversible kind) in order to avoid septic shock and relieve pressure at the point of the leakage. They had seen this before, my surgeon said. When he had done the original surgery, a lot of the tissue was "quite a mess." Likely due to the radiation. So maybe one of the staples couldn't get a good hold on the tissue, and hence the leak. Maybe it was a mechanical failure in the staple machine. The irony is that the abscess was about twice as large as the tumour they took out.

The colonoscopy, the doctors said, would prevent septic shock and let the infectious material escape. Then, they thought, the rupture would heal and the cavity that had been created by the leak would slowly shrink and disappear. At least that was the idea.

For me, however, the immediate issue was pain. Excruciating pain. It felt like that form of torture described in the history of the Inquisition wherein a red-hot metal pole was inserted into a certain orifice.

This was quite different from my first surgery when the pain was well controlled by intravenous opiates. Now, however,

I was dealing with chronic pain that was not on a diminishing slope. Afterwards, my surgeon readily admitted he had little pharmacological experience with this kind of situation – he really didn't know what range of drug treatments would be best. I was put on a hospital regime of tightly-controlled pain pills (not intravenous, which works much faster) and the dosage could only be changed by the surgeon when he visited every other day. As a result, I spent some of the worst nights of my life during 15 days in hospital.

I would never let that happen again. I am now aware that I do not have a low pain threshold, as I thought I did. In fact, I tolerate pain quite well. But there is no reason to tolerate it. It gets in the way of healing. If I ever end up in the hospital again, I will insist on the appropriate level of pain relief.

I got home July 18th after two weeks of getting increasingly stir crazy. At this point my medication was a combination of five drugs - two opiates (one a patch, the other a pill), an anti-inflammatory, a drug for damaged nerves, and Tylenol. It worked pretty well, though the side effects were dizziness, light headedness, sleepy periods, constipation, cold sweats, muscle tightness, and a wee bit of mental confusion (I can hear friends saying *Hey Bob, that's just you*).

So, I was at home with the assurance that doctors had seen this before, that the body would slowly absorb the matter in the cavity near my tail bone, and everything would slowly shrink, and close, and go away. Then everything would be fine.

That was the current plan.

And in the following months I have to say that it looked like we got the cancer. My enzyme tests (every three months) kept turning up negative (and this was the critical period, the first two years after surgery, when most cancers return). On the cancer front, things look good.

According to CT scans the abscess did start to shrink – during the first two months after surgery it went down by about a third of its original size. It looked like we were on course. I was at home, on long-term disability, and on a regime of pain management I had never known before. My main drug, *Dilaudid*, was a synthetic morphine that is about five times more powerful than morphine and three times stronger than oxycodone. It can lead to an addiction, but the doc says "let's call it 'dependence' and worry about it later."

So, most of the time I was not in great pain, maybe just a bit of discomfort. But if I was late with a dose, the pain returned with a vengeance. So there was always this nagging **fear of pain**.

More troublesome were the side-effects – the dizziness, nausea, woolly-headedness, cold sweats and muscle rigidity. And as my body grew accustomed to the drugs there was a growing **tolerance** for the opiate – so I had to take more, and that meant more side-effects. I switched to *Fentanyl* (a synthetic about 60 times stronger than morphine gram for gram – though you take very little) with *Dilaudid* as a break through relief.

But I managed all this with the belief that the abscess was shrinking and all would soon be well. I was walking in the sun and I think I had the best tan since I was a teenage camp councilor. My mom scolded me that I looked better than I felt - and that's no way to get good sympathy.

By mid-October, a CT scan showed that my post-surgery abscess was about one-third the size it was when I left hospital. The pain, however, had not shrunk in tandem with the abscess. Still, I was hopeful. We would get to January, 2008, and then reverse the colostomy, and everything would be fine.

Or not.

I was on the examination table in early January when my surgeon pointed to the TV monitor to show that the leak in the rectum was still open. It had not healed. That meant they could not reverse the colostomy. And it could mean the pain would be permanent.

I was coming to realize that, at least in my case, there are worse things than cancer.

I have been given the option of living with the current pain (and the discomfort and difficulty of a colostomy) or re-doing the entire surgery. And as of this writing I am going for the latter option. Mostly because otherwise I have to live with synthetic morphine and side-effects that dull the brain and body. Not what I would want for another 20-30 years of life where I think I can contribute many things in broadcasting and music and family and community. So … here we go again. Surgery impending.

Through all of this, I am mindful of so many good friends who have shared much of their lives, big chunks of their time, the fullness of their prayers, and the warmth of their hugs to help me in this struggle.

And to Frances and Michael – always my love.

Jennifer Baker

Ottawa, Ontario.

Brain cancer

———■———

My journey began one fateful Friday the 13th in June, 2003 when I collapsed suddenly at work from a grand mal seizure. I was rushed to the hospital and 11 days later I underwent brain surgery to remove a massive tumour from the right side of my brain. Pathology tests revealed my worst nightmare - a grade 3 Astrocytoma Oliogodendroglioma. In layman's terms - Brain Cancer!

Sadness, fear, and a child-like helplessness are all words that only touch the surface of what I felt upon hearing the word CANCER. To make matters worse, I had no family nearby to support me as I faced an uncertain future. But, I firmly concluded that I had to be strong and not let this disease envelop me.

Within weeks of my surgery, I endured six weeks of daily radiation treatments. This caused some hair loss, but my fashion sense took over, and I scoured the malls for stylish hats, as surgery left my head too sensitive to wear a wig. Additionally, I took specialized chemotherapy pills for brain cancer, five days each month for a year. I battled nausea, and a horrific bout of depression which had me, at times, overwhelmed with thoughts of suicide. Oddly, I found solace in the comfort of my 3 cats who loved me bald, sick, and depressed. My love for them and their unconditional love for me made me realize that cancer was only a part of my life; it was not my whole life. So, I soldiered on.

To my dismay, some of my closest friends shunned me, perhaps out of fear. Yet others, who were mere acquaintances, came to my much needed aid. They took me out for meals, helped with groceries, and cheered me up when I was down. Even the neighbourhood chipped in with baked goodies, fresh fruit and invites for dinner. I had developed a surrogate family of friends who today remain my anchor in life.

Recuperation was endless, so to keep fit and maintain some semblance of sanity, I began walking. I marvelled at the fact that each walk netted me some loose change found on roads and sidewalks. In conjunction with this, I noticed a multitude of wild pansies had suddenly appeared throughout my entire property. Was this a sign? Since I was struggling with depression, I bought a book on angels to help cope with my spirituality. To my astonishment, I read: "How your angels communicate with you – through coins and a special flower". My dear mother had passed away in 1996 and her favourite flower was the pansy. I no longer felt quite so alone.

After 16 months, I returned to work part-time. But, once back full-time, my company let me go. This couldn't be any worse than getting Cancer, I thought. As I left the office for the last time, I found a dime!

It took me years to fully recover physically and emotionally. The surgery and cancer treatments left me with chronic headaches, insomnia, depression and even mild seizures. I was often overcome with fatigue and I'd lost my desire to work along with my overall zest for life. When I spoke of these debilitating symptoms to my doctors, they simply pulled out their prescription pads to load me with more pills which always made me feel worse. Finally, I took control and sought help from a nutritionist who opened my eyes to enjoying good health the natural way.

Today, I still go for regular MRI's, and 5 years later have been given a clean bill of health by my Oncologist. I study nutrition endlessly, particularly the role of balancing the body's pH to prevent and fight disease. I attend monthly support group meetings and try to be an inspiration to others inflicted with this dreadful disease. Volunteer work for both the Brain Tumour Foundation and an animal rescue organization allows me to give back to those that helped me through my journey.

In the beginning, I was terrified of recurrence, but with time came healing, both physical and emotional and now, I feel healthier and happier than ever. Although I realize life can be taken away very suddenly, I have a new appreciation for the life I could have lost. There are no more bad hair days, and small annoyances are less annoying. Life is good and Cancer is only a mere chapter in my wonderful book of life.

Alice McClymont

Ottawa, Ontario

Breast Cancer, lobular invasive.

———————— ▪ ————————

S ix years ago, at the age of 55, I got a call that all women fear after having a mammogram. I was told a small lump was showing up and I would have to have a biopsy to determine whether it was benign or cancerous. My GP said he would call before the weekend, so when I had not heard, I was quite sure the news was not good. I called him back while at work on a small consulting job with a government department. I had prepared myself for bad news so was not surprised when he said that unfortunately the lump was malignant and I was being referred to a surgeon at the Women's Breast Health Centre at the Civic Hospital. I remember calling my husband, Ian, who wanted me to come home immediately. I felt quite calm and wanted to finish my day and my contract which was ending later that month. I suggested my husband come down for lunch which he did, and I think it helped him deal with it when he saw how calm I was. I also remember that when I told one of the women on the team at work, she had tears in her eyes.

Then the process of dealing with breast cancer began. The whole experience had so many positive moments that they outweighed the negative and actually left me feeling more full of life, and with more appreciation of how precious each day is, and how important my family and friends are to me. The surgeon I was referred to was Dr. Mark Hardy and he was a tremendous help in getting me through the experience with his professional manner and excellent skills, but just as importantly with his patience, gentleness and sense of humour. I always looked forward to our meetings with him, and Ian also spoke very highly of him.

When I had my surgery for a lumpectomy, he was there before the surgery and actually walked with me to the operating room. I was fortunate to have Stage 1 breast cancer which was lobular invasive, the stage being determined by the size of the lump, the grade and the fact that there was no lymph involvement. I did have many lymph nodes removed during the surgery which has compromised my lymph system and I have to be more careful of my right arm, a small price to pay when I found out that all the lymph nodes were clear and I would not have to have chemo. Being told I would have 25 radiation treatments was much less scary and I handled them with only some tiredness as side effects.

The night before my surgery I had a visitor, a woman from Victoria' Quilts who presented me with a beautiful quilt made by my friend Missy who is one of the volunteers with this group who make quilts for cancer patients. What a fabulous service. The one night I was in hospital after surgery I felt great, had several visitors from the family and two women from my book club who brought a basket with fun gifts including a book.

The surgery was February 13 and as I was to be in hospital and recovering over Valentine's Day, Ian declared Valentine's Day early for us that year and whisked me off to Merrickville the week before for a surprise overnight. As I had finished my contract I decided not to worry about work for a while. In March with an okay from the doctors, Ian, Lauren, (our daughter) and I went to the Dominican Republic for a week. I remember shopping for a bathing suit without wires so that I would be gentle to my surgery site and we had a wonderful holiday. After my radiation treatments in April, again with the doctor's approvals, Ian and I went on a 2 week planned vacation tour to Greece and Turkey and I enjoyed every minute of it.

My follow up was with my oncologist Dr. Keller and he decided I was to go on tamoxifen for 5 years. So the cancer was gone, but as with all breast cancer there are no future guarantees and life goes on. Except for my yearly meetings with the surgeon and the oncologist, I put my experience behind me, but being cognisant of the fact that I had gone through a life-threatening illness and seeing each day as an opportunity to enjoy the small pleasures of life, to appreciate my family and friends, and to plan interesting outings and trips.

In October 2002, I walked the 5 km walk with my two daughters, Tanya and Lauren and raised money for breast cancer. My reminders of that walk are that I won several prizes for the amount I raised, including a suitcase with the breast cancer logo, an umbrella and a cap and scarf. A colleague that I had worked with who found out about my cancer mentioned that there was a dragon boat team of breast cancer survivors and I should check it out. Not being a strong swimmer and never being on a sports team, I didn't think this was for me, so resisted until she mentioned it again when we met a couple of years later. So in 2005 I attended an orientation at Breast Cancer Action and went out to the Rideau Canoe Club one evening in May to try out practice paddling. It was a lovely warm evening and I met some lovely women and after being fitted for a lifejacket, got into the boat with 19 other paddlers, a drummer and a steersperson and the coach. I was hooked.

Joining the dragon boat team was one of the best decisions of my life. The enjoyment and support I have had from the team, the paddling and the festivals is more than I could have imagined. My first year paddling, our team won the Breast cup in Stratford which was a thrill for someone who had never competed on any team before. As well as the paddling in the summer and the opportunity to go to festivals in Canada and internationally, the team also trains during the rest of the year, doing aerobic exercises, circuit training, running, walking and pool paddling to get ready for the festival season. In June 2006, I celebrated my 60th birthday and decided to have a big party. Approximately 80 people helped me celebrate in my backyard and in lieu of gifts, many gave donations towards my trip with Ian to the International Breast Cancer Dragon boat Festival in September 2007. That trip was realized and will never be forgotten, as close to 40 women and many supporters from the Ottawa team travelled to Australia together and went on to tour Australia and New Zealand. There were over 2000 participants and many Canadian teams and being in the parade made us feel like we were at the Olympics. Ian and I stopped off in Fiji for a cruise on the way back.

In December 2007, I noticed that my right breast where I had had the breast cancer was changing. It was shrinking and becoming lumpy. I was concerned, but as it was close to Christmas and as I had a mammogram scheduled in January 2008, I decided to wait for the mammogram. The mammogram didn't show anything specific, but due to the changes I was sent for an ultrasound followed by an MRI. The MRI is much more detailed and showed a lesion in the right breast and some activity in the bones.

My oncologist was in contact with my GP and they were puzzled by the fact that I had no pain in the bones, so were not completely sure at this point that the bone activity was cancer. I was then sent for a biopsy and a bone scan. The biopsy showed a definite lesion in the breast which was lobular invasive cancer like last time, but larger and more aggressive and the bone scan kept showing activity in certain areas that appeared to be cancer.

Following the biopsy, I started having pains in my back, but thought they were the result of the biopsy. The oncologist referred me to a surgeon. Unfortunately, Dr. Hardy had left Ottawa last year so I had to change surgeons, but was very happy with my referral as I had heard good stories from many of my dragon boat friends about him. However, the meeting did not go as expected, as the surgeon was convinced based on the tests that my cancer had metastisized to the bones and that I should be treated for this before he did any surgery for the breast. This was my first real shock as I had to face the fact that it looked as though I did in fact have Stage 4 breast cancer, which is when the breast cancer metastisizes. It was also a shock not to go through surgery first as this was what I had expected. For the first time I broke down and felt afraid and nervous. It was such a comfort to have Ian with me. That evening I started to announce my news to my choir and broke down again as the news was so fresh in my mind. However, since then I have not shed tears; in fact have shed more tears over the fact that my son Jake's beloved Bassett had to be put down after he developed cancer in his lung.

Following a CT Scan, I had a long meeting with the oncologist who verified that I did indeed have cancer in the bones, in the sternum and in the spine. His opinion was that it was a new primary and the treatment he outlined was three forms of chemo and a bone strengthener to start March 14 and be administered every 3 weeks for 6 sessions.

So began my chemo journey at the General Hospital. My first session went well, the nurses were very gentle and kind, the patient in the next bed was a very positive glamorous young woman, my veins were good for the IV, Ian was with me for the full 5 hours and we got through it. I went home exhausted.

The next two days I took many pills, including a steroid which kept me energized to the point that I attended a St. Patrick's Day dance at my church and danced the jive and the polka with lots of energy left over. The home visiting nurse came twice and helped to reassure me that everything I was experiencing was normal but to watch out for fever and sudden pain. I had taken the next week off work and just read and dozed and talked to friends and felt so lucky that I wasn't sick and that my only side effect was tiredness which was very normal particularly during the time that the white blood cell count goes down.

The second and third weeks I was back to work and to my other activities such as exercise, choir, going out with friends and book club.

My second chemo treatment was on April 4. There were two minor glitches in that my blood count was too low the day before so I had to take another blood test and didn't know for sure if the chemo treatment was going to go ahead till the last minute, but it did and the nurse had trouble getting the IV into my veins, but finally did. The pattern held for the first week and my energy is back now in the second week.

Before starting my chemo treatment, I got my long hair cut short and then 2 weeks after the first treatment when it started to come out, I had it cut off and shaved into a buzz cut. I also got fitted for a wig in a shorter hairstyle, but in the same blonde colour I was used to. I like my new wig and have many comments on it with most people not realizing it is a wig. My family and friends like my buzz cut as well and I don't feel as self conscious about it as I thought I would. After all, it is just hair and it will grow back. My goddaughter was telling me about a young woman she knows who has alopecia and has to wear wigs all the time, so I feel fortunate that my hair will grow back. In the meantime, I have new looks. It helps that I look healthy and I smile a lot because every day good things happen. The woman in the bed next to me at my first chemo treatment had a very glamorous wig on and she looked great. I am thinking of getting another one with a more curly look like my own hair.

I am constantly amazed at how much love and support I am getting from so many quarters. Of course my husband Ian is my main support as my caregiver, driver, cook and cleaner, chemo buddy and the one who watches movies with me, talks to me and reminds me to drink more water and take my temperature and not to overdo it when my energy is back up. My children, stepchildren, step-grandchildren, goddaughter, Tracey and family, brother and sister are all there calling me, visiting, bringing food or inviting us for dinner, sending flowers, sending lots of emails and just showing me how much they love me. Tracey comes over to visit with her 10 month old son, Thierry, who brings me great joy. Three of my close girlfriends, Marcia, Ursula and Raymonde came for a visit and brought a gift of a lovely pink lingerie set. Two other friends, Don and Joan who live out of town came to cook for me. My neighbours have been supplying us with food and regular calls to see how I am doing. Each day I get cards in the mail, masses or novenas being said for me, candles being lit for me, and phone calls and emails from family and friends in Britain, Poland and the US, as well as Canada telling me how they are thinking of me. The members of my choir have also been my support and one of our priests will be doing a service for the healing of the sick during one of our choir practices later this month. My boss and colleagues at work have been amazing. I had not been in the job long before all my tests started and when it was confirmed that I had cancer and would have to have treatment, they could not have been more flexible with my work schedule and their constant support through flowers, cards and concern. This allows me to work when I can without feeling any pressure.

And then there is my dragon boat team who are a constant and very special support as they have all gone through breast cancer and some have gone through metastatic breast cancer. They are my heroes and my inspiration. I see some of them at exercise class, some at the Saturday morning walks, and many at functions such as potlucks, auctions, meetings and fundraisers. I look forward to paddling with them in May and at the festivals this summer. A couple of weeks ago one of the women from the team who is in charge of the Care Committee came by with a very large bag full of gifts from the team members. There were books, magazines, candles, writing paper, chocolates, bath stuff, a puzzle and many more surprises. Everyone going through a recurrence gets this treatment and it is a powerful incentive to keep going and stay positive.

It has been interesting to see who steps up to the plate in this type of situation. I have been very fortunate with so many supporters. There are still some negative surprises, friends who have not called or written and a family member who was not speaking to me and has not changed this stance in spite of the circumstances. These are hurtful, but so few in comparison to the many who have surpassed any of my expectations.

The changes I have made to my life are to concentrate on getting well, thus I am working less in my job, hardly working at all at home as I have the cleaning and cooking support, pacing myself with more rest, drinking much less wine, drinking a lot more water, and ensuring I get my exercise.

I hope I have a long life ahead of me, but in the meantime I look forward to reaching my short term goals, the next big one being June 27, my last chemo treatment, 2 days before my 62nd birthday. As stated in my title, this is just another stage. Last time I was Stage 1 and this time Stage 4. This is a scary jump and the literature is also very daunting. More stories need to be written about Stage 4, metastatic cancer that brings hope to those who get this diagnosis. This is one of them. Two of the women on the dragon boat team who have been particularly helpful to me are Mary O'Rourke and Chris Lynds, both of whom have also undergone a recurrence of breast cancer that has metastisized. For more information about them refer to Chris's blog at http://chris-theedgeoflight.blogspot.com

One of the things I would stress is that it is important to try and stay as stress free as possible during treatment. This is easier for those who are older and don't have young children and who have a lot of support. But there are still instances when stressful things happen that are surprising.

For the most part the medical people I have dealt with are excellent at being kind and compassionate but I have had a couple of unfortunate instances where I felt I was being treated with impatience and lack of compassion and this is hurtful when you are in treatment.

I also think that others who are dealing extensively with cancer patients such as those supplying wigs should be more compassionate and gentle. This is a time when a person is particularly sensitive and needs a lot of gentleness. An episode of not being treated well can stay with you and cause unnecessary stress.

Suggestions to relatives, friends and coworkers: I have been very fortunate in that most of my relatives, friends and coworkers have been very supportive and caring. To the others I would say you or someone you care about deeply may get cancer at some time and you will appreciate the concern and support of people. It doesn't take much to make a phone call or send an email or a card. If you have had a falling out with a relative or friend, now is the time to make the step to bridge the gap. Don't wait till it is too late. Just as the cancer patient gets inspiration from others, so those supporting the cancer patient can get much inspiration from how they are dealing with their illness.

There are always going to be some moments when you are feeling low but being able to pick yourself up and do something that gives you pleasure gets you out of that mood.

For new patients with breast cancer there are a lot of support groups and the Breast Cancer Action is a great place to call and get information or be put in touch with someone who has gone through it.

Beverly Maybee

Ottawa, Ontario

Leukemia

———————■———————

S itting in the Queensway Carleton emergency, assuming I'd had an allergic reaction, to being told several hours later you have leukemia (what shock, disbelief), to which I asked, so when can I go back to work? They looked at me in shock and said, "you don't seem to understand. You are basically walking dead". We hadn't even heard of the word leukemia in 1999, so we had no idea whatsoever what it was or how much our lives were about to change.

After a few hours of crying, shouting and just plain freaking out, you have to pull yourselves together. My husband (Dale) had to call England and tell my parents and family and also get a family history (of which there was and still is no mention of leukemia). I also had my daycare business, parents were counting on me, our dogs, my 3 step children then aged 8, 11 and 12, all these things in our lives had to be organized. You have to look forward and believe it is going to be alright. When Dale told everyone, it was one of the hardest things to do. No one knew what to do or say.

.My husband Dale was back then, and still is to this day, my tower of strength. I don't think people realize it, but it wasn't only me going through this horrible disease - the whole family was, as Dale had to do all the cooking, cleaning, banking, dogs, children to activities, groceries etc, and all while I am lying in a hospital bed trying to deal with my stuff.

I guess looking back now, there should have been a change in my outlook on life, but I was taught from a young age by my parents, no matter how bad things get for you, there is always someone else somewhere worse off than you, and that's the approach we took. I saw that the others who were diagnosed at the same time as me (about 6 of us all together I believe), I am the only one here today.

We found we had to change our lives a little as there were restrictions back then such as no malls, theatres, restaurants and most definitely no trips for at least 3 months (which turned out to be 8 years for the trips as you will see why later on), as you had to be close for daily hospital visits, and V.O.N visits. I had to reorganize my daily routine once back home as I couldn't stand up to cook which I loved to do, so I brought veggies etc to the table to chop, and sat, and did most of the meals from there, and then Dale cooked. You feel useless a lot of the time, as simple things like doing the laundry I couldn't even lift the basket, let alone take it down 4 flights of stairs to the laundry room, so someone had to do that. I would follow, put on a load and putter in the basement till it was done, then change it over and keep going. Then someone had to carry it all the way back up again so it could be put away (in our new house we have the laundry on the bedroom level). I couldn't even vacuum as I had a Hickman (this is a surgically implanted device in to the main artery to the heart which allows meds to be given and blood to be drawn) if while vacuuming or scrubbing floors it could come out and then you are in trouble.

I think one of the biggest impacts on my life was losing my daycare I had started several years earlier in our home. I have always worked with children. I was 16 years old when I became a nanny in England (which is where I was born), and came to

Canada in 1986 as a nanny then opened my daycare, wonderful families and all boys it was great.

Another thing would be how Dale and I had decided in 1999 to try to have a child of our own only to be told to wait and see how things went with treatments. Also how our friends didn't want to be around us. We think it might have been because so little was known about leukemia back then that they were afraid they might catch it or something, but even today there isn't much known about the disease itself which is hard to take in for me as there are so many people almost daily still being diagnosed with this disease which is a cancer as well.

I would like to let new patients of any cancer know that you should be positive at all times. When I was in the hospital I was known as the happy one (as I was always smiling even if I didn't feel like it as laughter and smiles make you and others around you feel better), and I was always doing things like, making tea/coffee or toast for the others, (even if I felt really bad I couldn't just lie in that bed). Doing these things MADE me get out of bed, and then I had Dale bring in craft supplies and started making clay ornaments, bead animals etc. So when I was not well they knew it. I learned to expect the unexpected, take one day at a time but still look forward, as all patients were back then and are to this day, different. DO NOT believe all you read. Please talk to your doctors for advice on where to go for information as there is so much out there which is untrue. You need to know if the information is written by a doctor who has had dealings with this disease, not just people saying what they have heard. Be very careful.

I believe our medical advice came from the best source, our B.M.T. (bone marrow treatment) doctors. They were a team and all knew what each other was doing to one person, but even they couldn't tell us everything as we are all different. They could tell you what "might" happen, but if something different happened, which it did on several occasions to me, they would learn for future patients. As for medications, they were and still are done by body weight and a lot of good guess work by the pharmacists as all our bodies are different. Think of it like a diet, too little doesn't work, too much and it could mean the difference between life and death (not a good way to lose weight any way).

We did do research, mostly Dale and friends, but as we said a lot of it was "BAD". Our doctors noticed what we were reading and gave us the best advice which was, look for work from qualified doctors or professors only, (still didn't understand the disease but a lot less reading to do). What you have to remember is back in 1999 there was very little known about LEUKEMIA let alone all the different types there were.

As for support groups back in 1999, there were none. I just tried recently and still no one can help. That is why I decided to take part in this book in the hopes to get LEUKEMIA out there for those who are being diagnosed as we speak. Even the breast cancer society didn't know what to do for me. There was a program called Beautiful Women, Beautiful Minds (I believe I got the name right) who did wigs and make up to help with the outside, but it was, and still is, the inside that is affected. And really back then the wigs itched like mad, especially in the summer. Unfortunately, it seems BREAST CANCER is still the most advertised cancer in the world even though 99% of cancer patients be it breast, colon, or leukemia we all have to do chemo, radiation or a combination of both, neither of which I would wish on anyone once let alone twice in 2 years.

I wasn't able to make the decisions on my medications or treatments. I didn't know anything about the disease and you are supposed to be able to trust your team of doctors (which we did and still do 9 ½ years later). I have tried several times over the years to lower my medication doses, to which I usually got G.V.H. (graft versus host issues), some of which were, dry eyes (had to have all 4 tear ducts plugged surgically as I couldn't produce tears at all and still can't so on tear drops always, didn't like that), my lungs were affected and now I only have a $1/3^{rd}$ the capacity plus the asthma. Then I got rapid cataracts (more eye surgery, REALLY disliked that and now have to wear bifocals, which is a pain), also had full body rashes as we found that I seemed to have a lot of bad reactions to drugs, so we tried again till we got it right. The worst drug for me then and still to this day is the steroids. They are great for keeping the body going but when you try to drop the dose that's when the graft versus host issues come creeping out, and here we go again (it sounds scary I know, and it was, and is, but hey I'M ALIVE).

Please remember that we are all different and what happened and is still happening to me, isn't necessarily going to happen to you or any one you know with leukemia. On my first bout of leukemia in 1999 I was very physically sick for days, lost my hair (which strangely enough NEVER bothered me, and besides my step children got revenge with the sunscreen, so there is a positive for every negative for someone), lost most of my upper thigh muscle control. Still to this day I can't kneel for long or stand, and after long walks my legs go wobbly, but you deal with it as best you can. Memory loss is hard to deal with, as is the weight loss. I lost half my body weight first time around. GREAT, but not the way to go (I was a heavy woman and still on the large side). I have also developed sleep apnea which they believe could be due to the transplant in 2000 (more on that later). Bone density is a big one as the steroids do a lot of damage so I have to do yearly scans for that (I have a little osteopeonia which considering 9 ½ years of prednisone that's good). I think the worst side effect to look at had to be losing all my finger and toe nails, yes you heard me right. They start from the base and kind of come forward then peel away. I know disgusting, but cool to see and yes they grew back, but they all have little lines all over them so nail polish is a challenge.

Other than doing coffee/tea and toast runs for those who I felt were in a bad way, I would do crafts. Dale would bring in my beads, clay supplies and I would just play at making whatever, and hand them out to the doctors, nurses and patients. It brought a smile to most of their faces, and even requests sometimes, which made me feel even better. Once out for longer than a weekend, I found I was watching TV a lot like the Rosie O'Donnell show (she made me laugh a lot, great therapy), cooking shows, (most of the time I fell asleep so I guess they helped with the resting part). The telephone was great as I got calls constantly, seeing if I needed anything, and making sure that I was alright. This made me feel good and that people did care.

I don't believe I have come to terms with the disease, as there was no one to explain what was going to happen, would I live or die? What was I going to go through? What are our lives going to be like? How do you tell the children? Things like that should be addressed at the beginning and continued throughout. I hope that this piece will get the word out and make people realize there needs to be a support group for LEUKEMIA patients and their families as well as other cancer support groups. I must admit though that doing this piece for your book was hard as I had to go back and open doors in my mind that I haven't ever talked about in the 9 ½ years. So this was hard but good therapy, very emotional for Dale and myself. I did, however, end up seeing a psychologist for a few weeks as I started to have nightmares and my doctors were thrilled about that, as they said I have NEVER dealt with all the things that have happened to Dale, family and myself, but once again that is because of the lack of information available to the patient and their families, at no fault of the doctors or nurses.

I don't really think there is a story to share with newly diagnosed patients to help them, but I would like them and their families to always remember these things: always be positive, trust your doctors, ask questions, and the one thing I never did and I guess I should have was do a journal. This is good for many reasons. Had I done one I wouldn't have to be thinking so hard for this piece. I could see when I was at my worst/best, how my meds did etc., this is a big one I think.

I will be honest with you all, I do worry about recurrence as I was re-diagnosed in 2000 late summer, almost 1 year later (they have noticed this happens a lot but not sure why). I had just returned from visiting my parents in England for there 40th anniversary, and did blood work at the hospital, got the call saying to come in (we knew something wasn't right), found out I had got a different type of leukemia and they were not sure how to treat me, so I told them, I'm British I have to be different. So I am going home and doing the Hope Volleyball that Saturday and when they had an idea to call me. They were not happy I know, but to sit in a bed and wait for days till they figured out what to do, NOT Me. So I did go to the Hope Volleyball (I did not play much). They decided I needed a stem cell transplant. The word TRANSPLANT is a very scary word when it is thrown at you out of the blue. So we started the search, and didn't have to look far as they asked about siblings. I have a sister 17 months older than myself, Sharon is her name. The first thing was to have my head doctor call her and get some information, then try to do most of the pre-testing in England (which with the doctors help here and good communication went well). She was a match 100%. You might be thinking that's great and it was, but she is the reason for the graft versus host problems (she had such strong white cells that when I tried to down the doses of medications I would get G.V.H. as fore mentioned). However, she did come over and go through so many tests, screenings etc, they found her a good candidate for the alo-transplant, so we were here, our parents in England very worried as you can imagine about they're two girls and not able to do anything but wait and hope. We both made it. I had to do chemo and 6 sessions of radiation in 3 days to kill me off as I call it, so they could bring me back to life (it's the easiest way to explain it I find). Sharon had to come in from our home in the west end (which was another thing Dale had to do by driving her then going to work) 3 days in a row and lie in a bed not allowed to move. I fed her jubejubes, got her water etc. The worst thing is that Sharon was and still is a smoker and she couldn't smoke in the hospital (she did get a few in during breaks though). I did get very upset when I saw her lying there as it really scared me and I remember crying and thinking that it could do damage to her and change her life, (she has 2 girls of her own to think about as well).

That is one thing I remember really well because it brought us closer than ever before and I owe my life to her and as you can see we made it. The best thing is they tell you after that you can take on the traits of the donor. Great, she smokes, drinks lager (yuck), is allergic to strawberries and snow, yes snow. We just laughed and I told her anything but those as I love strawberries, snow, don't smoke, not allergic to snow and I don't like lager (how different can 2 sisters be?).

If there was yet another recurrence I would like to think I would be more informed as it is almost 10 years since the last recurrence and there is more known now than then (still not enough). Would I react the same? Most likely as I am an emotional person any way and the first thing which has come into my head both times is "oh no what how will we manage" (money wise so as not to lose the house, car). I can't get insurance due to the leukemia so it is only Dale's income we have to rely on. I would do more of the resting and accept help when it is offered if there was a next time (I am very stubborn and don't like to accept what I would call charity), but I have learned it's not charity, it's help from concerned family and friends still hard to do, but it would take pressure off Dale and the family.

Since I have had a recurrence, and it was found on a regular blood work day, I would make sure I don't miss any appointments, rest up till they say what is to happen next and take all my medications. As for reacting, it is still a shock, you are scared, angry. I wasn't sure if I wanted to go through it again as it was going to be a more aggressive treatment regime (not just hard on me but Dale, family as well) and I still would like to know WHY ME? I still took the advice of my BMT doctors who were and still are very supportive and informative on what they would be doing. We knew we could and had to trust them.

YES, we did get support from both families and friends, even though mine were and still are all in England. We got a phone in the hospital and Mom and I talked everyday which made us both feel better. That was a life line for all of us. You find out who your friends are when something like this happens. We lost quite a few and we believe it was they really didn't know much about leukemia and it scared them off, but the ones who did come around are still in our lives and think we respect each other even more now. I don't get to see my sister much as she lives in England, but this has made us closer. We talk on the phone more and actually I can't imagine what was going through her head when we asked her to come all this way to help save her baby sister (we will always be grateful for that as we knew lots of patients who's family members had backed out at the last minute, so I am extremely lucky she gave me my life back).

Poor Dale was the one who had to tell everyone what was going on. When he called my parents my Mom answered and he started to tell her and she just said, "I don't want to talk to you", and handed the phone to my dad. He listened and was upset, and finally got Mom to tell Dale the family history. It was more that they were so far away more than anything and felt useless, and we wouldn't let them come over as it would have been too hard for them to go to and from the hospital every day, that is why the phone was the best thing we did (unfortunately the phone service is no longer free in the hospital which is a shame as long term patients don't have any other way to contact the outside world. This should be rethought). Dale's office co-workers were really understanding and he could come and go to visit me whenever. Back then he had 2 jobs so 7.30 am till 3.30 pm government job, then home grab a bite, (usually junk food), off to 2nd job at the race track in Quebec till midnight or later, then to see me, yes, that late. He was allowed because of his schedule, stayed half an hour then off home to start again, so now you see why he is my HERO. We did have to change the schedules and give up the 2nd job, especially when we got custody of his 3 children. To this day his office is still very supportive, (thanks to them all).

We may be ill, but we are not porcelain, so don't stop us doing things we can do, (within reason). We feel useless enough and that doesn't help us get mobile and on with our lives. You can't catch it, keep your life as normal as possible, drink lots of water as you don't want to dehydrate and end up on I.V.'s for 2 hrs as you have better things to do, but stay away from people who are sick as your immune system is none-existent.

Remember this most of all: THERE IS SOMEONE OUT THERE WORSE OFF THAN YOU.

I hope this is of help to anyone who has been newly diagnosed with leukemia, even if it helps one person that is one more than before. Good luck. Stay positive.

Thanks to all who have supported us through the years and those who have stuck it out, you know who you are.

Lynda Lubin

Montreal, Quebec.

Breast Cancer.

———————■———————

I received the diagnosis 3 hours after a more or less routine visit that I had breast cancer. I was 44 years old, with no family history of breast cancer. My initial reaction was that of complete shock.

I told no one about the diagnosis (except my husband) until it was confirmed 5 days later. I spent those 5 days very quietly. Once the diagnosis was definite. I dealt with it by regaining some sense of control. I decided that I was going to learn about the benefits of complementary health care so that I would know that I was being covered by conventional medicine as well as complementary.

My husband (I am since divorced) was a very good physical support. He drove me to appointments, he picked up food and prescriptions and helped with the children, but it was my kids, my family and friends that gave me the emotional support I needed.

I remember having an argument with my husband about my outlook on life. He thought that I should no longer care if the kitchen was tidy or if the beds were made, that I should just be happy I was alive. Of course I was happy to be alive, but I had always appreciated life and I wanted things to continue on as normally as possible.

I completely adjusted my diet. I became a vegetarian. I eliminated most dairy and wheat products as well. I stopped drinking coffee (I have since gone back to drinking 1-2 cups of organic coffee a day).

I also began to practice yoga soon after my chemo treatments ended.

I think the greatest impact was seeing cancer through the eyes of my children. At the time, my eldest daughter (Amanda) was 20, my son (Jesse) was 17 and my youngest daughter (Gabrielle) was 12.

Amanda took on the roll of caretaker. She immediately stepped up to the plate and decided she was going to take care of me, but at the same time she was going to do all she could to learn about prevention. She has subsequently become a holistic health counselor and yoga instructor.

Jesse, on the other hand, was a bit more distant. He would check in on me, and comment that I looked like GI Jane (thought the bald head was cool). Although I knew how much he cared, he basically stayed away most of the time. Recently, he mentioned that he could barely remember those few months.

Gabrielle's reaction was different than the others. She was much more concerned about whether or not I was going to die. She kept herself very busy socially. It was important for her to be busy all the time. She had the hardest time with my baldness, and for the first few months she wanted to make sure I was wearing my wig when her friends were around.

Today, almost 6 years later, my children are all very well adjusted and they never shy away from anyone with any kind of disease, chronic or otherwise. My cancer has made them stronger individuals. I am extremely proud of all of them.

I want people to know how very important it is to be an advocate for your own body. I was a "healthy" 44-year-old woman, with no history of breast cancer and no symptoms. When I asked for a routine mammogram, I was told that there was no reason to have one….I insisted on having one….I thank God that I did because that saved my life. I was told by the surgeon that because of where the tumor was located, that I probably would not have felt it for at least another year.

I was very fortunate to have been diagnosed at the Ville Marie Breast Center here in Montreal. They were thorough and I never had to wait for answers. I did send all my results to a doctor in The United States, and he completely agreed with the course of treatment.

I stayed away from the computer, but one of my best friends did a lot of extra research for me. When I was given a choice to be on a protocol or go with the traditional treatment, she called and spoke to one of the doctors who were leading a study in the United States. She compiled all the information and only showed it to me when I needed to make some very informed decisions.

There is a psychologist on staff at the center, and it was mandatory to see her before the surgery. We were also encouraged to bring a family member along. It was very helpful.

I was given a choice on whether or not to participate in the study or whether to have the traditional treatment. Before I made my decision, however, my case was presented to a tumor board (a group of doctors and specialists from several hospitals in the city). 10 out of 10 agreed with the protocol…well that made my decision very easy.

I experienced a lot of nausea and a lot of fatigue. I was very weak, but the worst symptom was that I could never find a place for myself. I was always coming out of my skin. I would doze off and wake with a start, disappointed to see I had fallen asleep for only a few minutes.

I also lost my sense of smell and taste, but that came back shortly after the chemo was finished. I walked and walked and walked some more. I would listen to Diana Krall when I was lying down.

I don't know that I ever came to terms with the disease, but eventually I was able to stop thinking of myself as Cancer…I was a person with cancer who was going to take control and do everything I could to fight .

I think anyone who has ever had any disease worries about recurrence. I continue to lead a healthy lifestyle. I exercise, I eat well and I try to keep a positive attitude.

My family and friends were a blessing. They intuitively knew when I needed them near me or when I needed to be left alone. To friends, family and co-workers I would like to say: please never ignore the situation. Acknowledge the cancer, acknowledge the fact that this is the fight of their life. You will know if they want to talk about it or not. If they do…great…be there to listen. If they don't, that is fine as well, but at least there will not be a white elephant in the room.

Send food, don't ask. If they have small children, offer to take them out for a bit.

I am a lucky, lucky woman.

Genevieve Pickett

Nepean, Ontario

Hodgkin's Disease, Stage 1A

———■———

I am a 31 year survivor of Hodgkin's Disease, in relatively good health and am very proud of having the privilege of seeing my four children grow up and getting to know my 5 grandchildren and watch them grow up. At the age of 32, when I was diagnosed, I was so scared that I would not live long enough to see my children grow up and that they would not have me there to make sure that they were taken care of by people who loved them. Determination and sheer luck or someone looking down on me from above helped me through the next five years when I was declared cured and throughout the future years when things cropped up because of the damage from the radiation treatment.

After two years of visiting my family doctor almost weekly to complain about the unbearable exhaustion, having been misdiagnosed twice, and living with a large lump in my neck for 9 months, I was finally diagnosed. My family doctor did not believe me and considered me physically and mentally exhausted because of a difficult family life I had at the time and possibly a thyroid disease. He advised me that it was a waste of time and money to refer me to a specialist for consultation. I had to almost blackmail him into making a referral which took about three months to materialize. I was finally diagnosed in a matter of a 10 minute consultation with a very astute endecronologist in St. John's, Newfoundland. The possibilities given to me during this visit were that I could have a benign tumor, a brachial cyst or cancer. I cried because I was relieved that someone finally believed that I was actually physically sick and that I was not losing my mind. I was not permitted to go home that day to prepare my family for the worst. I sat on a chair in a ward for a whole afternoon waiting for a patient to be discharged so that I could have a bed. It was a Thursday and I was already scheduled for surgery on Monday.

My primary concern at that time was the hope that I could live long enough to make arrangements to have my children taken care of by people who loved them. At the time my four children ranged in age between 2 and 11 years and we were living 400 km from the major health care treatment centre in St. John's. I spent seven weeks in hospital in St. John's (away from my children who could not visit me during that time) and underwent three rounds of surgery in the first three weeks. The first was to explore the lump in my neck and make a diagnosis. Three tumors were found and resulted in the removal of one large gland and two small ones. The second was to conduct an exploratory between my lungs, diaphragm and ovaries to determine if the cancer was spreading and resulted in the removal of my spleen. The third was a bone biopsy procedure which resulted in the removal of a quarter-size chunk of bone from the top of my pelvic bone. The outcome of all this was that I was diagnosed with Stage 1A Hodgkin's Disease with a 90% chance of a cure if I agreed to a massive round of cobalt (radiation) treatment.

In all, I underwent 20 high intensity cobalt treatments on my chest, neck and under my arms and 15 more less intensive treatments on my ovaries over the next three months. I spent another seven weeks in St. John's over that three months from Monday to Friday undergoing radiation treatments and then went home for the weekend where I called up enough strength (to this day, I cannot believe that I sustained this routine) to encourage and ensure my children that I would live, do a mountain of laundry, cook good meals for the children, clean up a very messy house and put things in order for my absence over the next week. I even drank sylicane to deaden the pain resulting from the radiation on my throat and esophagus so that I could swallow food and keep up my health during the treatments. I was bound and determined to not have my treatments delayed and interrupted because of failing health due to the side effects of the radiation.

After seven weeks in hospital and the start of one week of extensive cobalt treatment I was allowed to go home to see my children. I was so thin and sick looking (about 100 pounds compared to my normal 135) that people in the community and my children were convinced that I would not survive. The impact on my children of them not being able to see me and have me comfort them during the weeks of absence is another story. The complete exhaustion caused by the disease was nothing compared to the treatments and side effects which I learned to live with and count my blessings that I would live to see my children grown up and get to know my grandchildren.

Today, I enjoy good health, make sure I get flu shots and keep my pneumovax up to date. Since I was diagnosed, I raised my children almost alone, had the privilege to witness a growth of a quantum leap for three of them from a small Bay in Newfoundland to Bay Street in Toronto. I divorced the children's father and moved to Ottawa almost 18 years ago. I also earned a University Degree which took 18 years of part-time study while working full time in a very busy and challenging career in community social and economic development and raising my children. I just retired from the Federal Public Service and can now relax and enjoy the next 20 years of watching and enjoying my grandchildren grow up, exploring new parts of this great country and the world with my soul mate, do volunteer work and maybe learn some new skills or do something new that I always wanted to do or haven't learned yet that I wanted to do it.

Looking back over the last 31 years, my advice to anyone who feels that their physician and friends are not giving them the right advice is to stick in your heels, go the distance and even threaten if necessary to get referrals to the right specialists. I feel that having been given the second chance to survive because I was determined to find someone who believed in me, I have been able to fulfill my dream to experience and do all the things I wanted to do in life before I leave this world. I kept my optimism high, always believed that there is always a solution to the most challenging situations and I never gave up on anything or anyone. I am still followed up annually through reports from my family doctor to my oncologist at the Ottawa Cancer Clinic.

There is a lot more to this story and I will be very happy to share it if it helps someone else understand that cancer can be beaten if you believe it and listen to your own body and take charge of your health. There are worse things than cancer which cannot be overcome as easy. Losing a loved one through tragedy and learning to live with the impact of loss of limbs, sight or living as a vegetable resulting from tragedy could be much worse to cope with.

Shirl Kennedy

Nepean, Ontario

Breast Cancer, metastatic stage

—————■—————

My breast cancer was detected on a mammogram in December 2003. I had a history of fibro adenomas for almost 20 years so when I felt this particular lump, I didn't run to my doctor in a panic like usual. I guess my lumps had cried "Wolf" too many times. Besides, I had a mammogram scheduled for December so when I first felt the lump in the summer, I waited until December to have it checked out.

For some strange reason, I had this notion that because I was having regular mammograms that it was preventing me from getting breast cancer. I thought no way could I possibly get breast cancer. After all, I had no family history of it. I ate a healthy diet. I didn't smoke, drink coffee or alcohol. I was getting regular mammograms. I had little stress as I had retired in 1997. I exercised daily … but surprise!!! I had breast cancer.

My first reaction was that I had six months to live. My minister was the first person to arrive when the news got out and she listened to me talk about death for 2 hours straight. It seemed the only women I knew with breast cancer had died but when I thought about it further I started to think of some who had survived the disease. I proceeded to call all of them to hear their stories. One of them, upon hearing my news, had a book on the subject (The Intelligent Patient Guide to Breast Cancer by Ivo Ollivotto MD, Karen Gelmon MD, and David McCready MD) and arranged to have it delivered to my door the same day which was a Friday. I was scheduled to see a surgeon on the following Monday. Over the weekend, I read the book and got a quick education about breast cancer and what to expect.

A biopsy ultrasound had been done which reported that the cancer had progressed to the lymph nodes under my arm. After my mastectomy, the pathology report said that 2 of the 20 lymph nodes removed were 'involved' so I was considered at 2nd or 3rd stage of cancer. My surgeon assured me that he felt that he had removed all of the cancer.

When the radiation oncologist said that I needed 25 treatments to kill any cancer cells that might still be in the area, I complied. Then, when my medical oncologist suggested 6 chemotherapy treatments, I hesitated. However, when she said that you get one chance to kill cancer and that is at the primary stage so let's hit it with both barrels (radiation and chemo), I agreed.

When my hair grew back, I started to dance through life again. I had my breast reconstructed so I could feel whole again. I stepped up my exercise program and started a new regimen from a book called "The Path to Phenomenal Health" by Sam Graci that included a diet of high protein, low sugar, fresh fruit and vegetables and essential vitamins. That same year, I started to experience a sore shoulder. My medical oncologist sent me for a bone scan to see what was going on. When the results came back, you can imagine my shock to find that my breast cancer had spread to all the bones in my torso. A couple of days later, when I felt some pain under my rib cage, an ultrasound was done and 6 tumours were found in my liver. I was now at fourth stage of cancer. This was in January 2007. Due to the condition of my bones – 2 vertebrae have been badly eaten away with the cancer and my right hip bone could fracture very easily – I decided to stop doing my daily power walking. And it`s especially scary trying to walk in winter in case I slip on the ice.

2007 ended up being a grueling year to say the least. I had to visit the hospital 60 times due to oncologist visits, another round of 9 chemotherapy treatments, 6 radiation treatments, an MRI, numerous CT Scans, an Ultrasound, an Echocardiogram, heart scans, port-o-cath problems and for other related symptoms.

So after all that, how am I coping with the challenges of living with cancer? Well, through all of this adversity, I was blessed to have great support from my husband, a few family members, friends, neighbours and my church family. We moved to a new house, a gorgeous Minto bungalow. I continue to enjoy singing in the choir and going to my prayer group meetings. I credit my good attitude to God being in my life. I pray every day with my next door neighbour. Also anybody who knows I have cancer prays for me, too. God gives me strength and hope and no fear. I believe that if it is His will, I will be cured of this cancer. All the results of the tests have been encouraging. My bones are improving and the tumours are shrinking. I believe all the positive outcomes are the result of God's healing touch.

One promising scientific discovery that also gives me hope is a drug that I am taking called Herceptin. Basically, it won't let the cancer cells divide. It only works on breast cancer patients whose tumours are HER-2 marked. The blessing is that I have that marking. Only about 20% of breast cancer patients have this marking. When I was at the primary stage of my cancer, this drug was only being given to those at the metastatic stage (fourth stage). In 2005, Ontario committed funding for Herceptin. It is now given at the primary stage along with chemotherapy; consequently, it is resulting in almost no recurrence.

My chemo treatments ended in August 2007 but I continue to receive bone strengthener and Herceptin every third Wednesday at the Cancer Clinic at the General campus. I am hopeful that I will survive this.

Joanne Lalonde

Ottawa, Ontario.

Breast Cancer, Triple-Negative Inflammatory

——————— ■ ———————

I am 45 years young and I am the youngest of my family of 4 girls. My Mother passed away of Breast Cancer back in 1985, she was only 47 years old. When we finally found out that she had Cancer it was too late, nothing could be done to save her. We were told that she would have about 3 months to live and that's exactly what happened, almost to the day. It was such an awful thing for us to go through, it was like someone punched us in the stomach and took our breath away. It happened so quickly, we felt totally useless because we couldn't help her, all we could do was to be with her and try to make her feel comfortable and try to ease the pain to make it easier on her. There was nothing anybody could do to stop it.

I have always had a big chest with lots of cysts and because of this and my mother's history of breast Cancer, I am always checking my breast and have regular Mammograms. In February 2007 I found another lump (cysts) in my left breast, I met with my family doctor and he made an appointment for me to have a removal. I also had an ultrasound test done as well because my breasts are very dense. The Hospital and my doctor confirmed that they could only see cysts and that there was nothing to worry about. But this time they felt different, the cysts were painful, hard, hot to the touch and they were growing. My doctor still insisted that the mammograms confirmed that it was only cysts and gave me anti-inflammatory medication for this. After 2 months of taking the pills nothing had changed, I was done listening to him and told him that I know my body and that this felt very strange to me. My gut feeling was telling me that something was very wrong (never doubt your gut feeling) so I pushed my doctor to refer me to a specialist. Well, that took another 2 months because they are so busy, so I suffered with the pain until I met with him. When he finally saw me, he seemed to agree with my doctor that they were indeed cysts and because my left breast was so much bigger my right one because of the growth, he suggested that I undergo a breast reduction so that both breasts would look the same. About a week before the surgery I noticed that I had a lump under my left arm, in my armpit and mentioned this to him. He said he would check into it when I have my surgery. So 2 months later in July, I was scheduled for my breast reduction and cysts removal. Surgery went well but a couple of days later I could still feel a hardness in my left breast as well as under my armpit. This totally freaked me out. I was thinking why didn't he remove all of those cysts, and what if I have to get more surgery. I don't know if I could go through this again...so I waited to ask these questions when I met with him 2 weeks later for my follow-up visit.

I showed up for my follow-up visit and to have the staples removed and that's when he told me that he had taken a biopsy and that the result was Cancer. You can imagine my reaction when he told me, I was in shock because I couldn't hear him anymore, all I could think about was my Mom and how scared I was that I might die just like her. My boyfriend Dave and I couldn't believe it, this is wrong, they've got it wrong, I do all the right things, I don't smoke, I try to eat healthy and I exercise on a regular basis, how can this be happening to me? I was feeling sorry for myself and saying why me and then all I could think about is how am I going to tell this news to my 18 year old son Martin, my sisters and my father.

Once I was over the shock I got very angry, I get mammograms done every year if not more, I even had an ultra-sound done, how can they have not seen this before? If the methods don't work for detecting these cancers why use them? All they could tell me was that mammograms and ultrasound machines have a hard time seeing anything if you have dense breasts. Well, if they don't work as well on dense breasts why use them? Isn't there anything else out there that would work better? So, we do have some technology but it could be much, much better. Maybe MRI's would be better suited for dense breasts. My surgeon made the necessary arrangements for me to meet with a Specialist at the Women's Breast Health Clinic. I met with him and he explained the kind of Cancer I was dealing with. I have what they call a Triple-Negative Inflammatory Breast Cancer. He said that it made him think of a Lamborghini because it is very exotic, fast, aggressive and rare and that they would have to deal with it right away. But unlike my mother's diagnosis I was never told that nothing could be done, quite the opposite, there are a lot of new treatments and techniques that could be done now. Let me tell you, within 3 weeks I was scheduled for a whole bunch of tests; bone scan, cardiac scan, abdomen ultrasound, chest x-ray, just to ensure that the cancer hadn't spread anywhere else and that it was only in the left breast and in the lymph nodes under my left arm. Once all the tests were done. I then met with my Medical Oncologist to decide what kind of treatment would work the best on my kind of cancer. He suggested that I would need Chemo, Radiation and eventually a Mastectomy. I was so blown away from all this info that I couldn't keep my head on straight, but my doctor looked me in the eye and assured me that we could do this and that we will beat this and this put my mind at ease. He also told me that it would be in my best interest to take a leave of absence from work for a year because of the severity of the cancer and the means to handle it. It would be very hard on my system and he didn't want me to be in an environment that might jeopardize my outcome. This also upset me because I am a very social, busy, outgoing person and I couldn't imagine myself being idle at home for that long.

My treatment is called TC - Taxol and Carboplatin and is very effective to treat triple negative inflammatory breast cancer. My doctor gave me some information sheets on these medications which I researched some more on the web. I also found some very helpful info on the Breast Cancer.org site. My oncologist did suggest that I take the Chemo course so that I would know what to expect. Well let me tell you...I found the course very helpful but scary at the same time. They tell you what to expect, the side effects you may experience but that not everybody has the same reactions. The list just went on and on and I found it all too much for me to take, I was really scared. They then give you a tour of the Chemo rooms and that really freaked me out as well because so many people have cancer, the rooms were full. I came home and cried for a while as this was so overwhelming for me. I couldn't think that I could go through this, this is too tough, how can I handle doing this every 3 weeks for 8 treatments, I'm just not that strong. Once I was calmer I discussed it with my boyfriend and figured out my options, I either have the treatments and get better or I don't and I could die from it....So I chose to live and give it my all. So I started the Chemo and because of the type of Chemo I have, I need to take medications to counteract the effects of the Chemo. So, the day before Chemo I start and keep taking pills for up to 5 days after my Chemo treatment to prevent serious side effects. I found these to be very helpful and for that I am truly lucky. The effects that I still experience from Chemo are, of course, hair loss, loss of taste buds, ringing in my ears, occasional heartburn, sore joints and fatigue. I also get some side effects from the medications that help me with the Chemo, in my case I am very prone to constipation so I have to take other medications to help me while I am taking these. All in all I find that I am very lucky with my side effects compared to the other stories I have heard. My wish is that I didn't have to go through all of this but at least this way it worked out for me.

While I was going through all of this, what helped me the most was my family and friends. I know that there are all kinds of support groups out there willing to help, but I just couldn't do it, I didn't feel comfortable talking to strangers even if they went through similar situations. I guess in a way, I just wanted to keep it to myself. I would just talk to my friends and family, they may not have known how to help me and what to say but just having someone listen and to let me vent did a world of good. What I did find helpful for me was that I could talk to my friends about how I was feeling, but then I wanted to hear what was happening in their lives and I would live vicariously through them. It was fun to hear all about the drama, excitement that they were dealing with. I was surprised to hear from different people that they thought I was really strong going through all of this. I never really thought of myself that way, I just do what I have to do. Also, for me, because I had to take a leave of absence from work, I had to apply for disability insurance. I found that my insurance company was and is continuing to be very helpful and supportive. I am so lucky to have such a good service available to me. I don't know how I could have handled all of the expenses without them.

They say that when the hard times come, that's when you can tell who you can count on and how much you are truly loved. I found that I am truly blessed with such good family and friends, you never really know how much until something like this happens. My friends and family really pitched in when I needed them. I had friends offer to bring in food, give me rides to appointments, take me out for walks and I found this very touching and I did take them up on their offers. The part that I found very difficult was with my pride, I would not let my friends and family clean my house. I am used to doing everything myself and I just couldn't let them do it for me, but that's just the way I am. We all have our hang-ups my family calls it being stubborn, oh well! I found that some people in my group of friends and family just couldn't handle the fact that I had cancer, they found all kinds of excuses not to come and see me (afraid to give me a cold etc.) and would never know what to say on the phone, they didn't want to call me in case I was sleeping or something. They even had trouble saying the C word. For these people I just let them be, I didn't want to force my situation on them. I know it can be scary, some people handle things differently, I don't hold any grudges.

In January I had my Mastectomy and everything went well and my surgeon confirmed that the pathology report did not show any traces of cancer in my left breast, nor in my lymph nodes. I am in remission right now. He seemed to think that the Chemo had done it's job at killing the Cancer, so for preventative measures my Oncologist wants me to finish with my 2 last chemo sessions to ensure that all the necessary precautions have been taken into consideration because of the type of cancer I have. They are not sure what the stopping point should be and that we do not want a relapse!

We are now in February, I have had 7 Chemo treatments up to now with one more to go, hopefully my last will be on March 12th. Right now I am still thinking about what is going to happen next; last Chemo, Radiation and as for reconstruction surgery, I don't know...so many things to think about. Do I want to go through more surgery? Can I live happily with just one breast? What are the pros and cons? All I know is that I don't have to decide this all now, I have time and it will come to me I'm sure. I still want to get more information on the web about these procedures and I also have a lot of books that my friends and family have given me for information.

As for recurrences, I don't want to think about that right now because I am still in the thick of it. Once I get the green light that everything is A-OK, then maybe I will start thinking of a recurrence (not that I would ever want that to happen). I want to put all of this behind me and concentrate on living my life the best way I know how. I want to do the things I like, get off the couch

and get active, experience things that I have
want to take life for granted anymore. They sa
the same after you've experienced something
It's like starting over from scratch, a do-over. `
that were wrong or the things you wanted to cha
can do it. I am up to the challenges ahead of m
doesn't kill you makes you stronger...and it's so true.

Well, the last of my 25 Radiation treatments finished in May.
I was very surprised at how tired I was after each treatment, I was
wiped out. I had a little reaction to the treatments it gave me a
rash, red, itchy bumps everywhere that I was treated. They went
away after of couple of weeks or so with the help of a prescribed
cream.

I agree that Breast Cancer is scary and it will turn your world
upside down but there is a lot of new information, treatments,
techniques that can make your life easier. You are not alone and if
you want and need outside support there are so many good people
who can help. You can find them through your doctors and nurses,
at the Cancer Centre, through the internet at Cancer.ca, so many
books out there etc. It doesn't have to be a scary thing.

How I cope with living with Cancer, well I live one day at a
time, glad that I am done with all the treatments for now. I try to
stay positive and have a good attitude and I try not to sweat the
small stuff. My boyfriend Dave and my son Martin take very good
care of me, I am so grateful to have them, I love them so much.
I have my family and lots of wonderful friends that help, support
and pray for me, in that regard I am very lucky. I look forward to
going back to work and seeing all my colleagues. I tell myself that
I have too many things that I haven't done or seen yet. I would
love to travel and visit Paris, Australia etc.. I would like to learn to
play tennis. I want to skydive (tandem). I want to eventually see
my son get married some day and have kids of his own. So, with
everything said and done, I try not to think of all the bad stuff
that comes with being sick with Cancer and the process of going
through it all but, rather I think of the things I will be able to do

...ent through all of this and for that I am truly grateful ...nother day.

I just want to take a minute and thank my Medical Oncologist for finding the right Chemo treatment for me and not treating me like a number. I also want to thank my Surgeon and the army of doctors, nurses, staff at the Cancer Centre if not for all of them I wouldn't be here today. Thank you!

A hopeful future Cancer Survivor!

Lois Rouble

Nepean, Ontario

Breast Cancer

———————■———————

In May of 1990 I was diagnosed with breast cancer. I was a single parent with 3 children still at home aged 22, 20 and 16. I was still going to Carleton U. to finish my degree and worked as a teacher by day. My youngest son has and still has a learning disability so he required quite a bit of assistance with his assignments as I was his editor.

My surgery resulted in a mastectomy and I was told to go home and enjoy life as the lump was encapsulated and I wouldn't require any further treatment.

The following February I had a breast reconstruction which was fine.

In Sept. 1991 I had a heart attack from stress. I was later diagnosed with a generalized distress disorder.

1994 came and in May I noticed a lump in the same breast as before but this time in the scar tissue. I wasn't as lucky this time as my cancer was invasive. Another surgery followed by 35 radiation treatments and 5 years of tomoxophin. I only missed 2 days of work for my treatments as I figured it was better to stay busy.

Then came 4 years of the principal from Hell. Needless to say my blood pressure was very high for these years. This principal had a history of trying to destroy teachers that she didn't like. I have been trying to forgive her for cutting short my wonderful career as a teacher. I think I finally have.

1999 brought about another problem. This time I had to have a hysterectomy because the walls of the uterus were thickening as a result of the Tomoxophin. Surgery went fine until my bowels froze and I couldn't eat, toot or poop. 23 days later with daily visits from my kids and family I was finally able to go home. From January on I could only work half time because I didn't heal very well. This time I was pre-cancerous.

Come, September with a new principal, she gave me another split grade a 4/5. I still wasn't very well. So in March after 25 years of teaching I had to go on Long Term Disability (LTD). What a joke, LTD is only for 2 years after you have used up all sick leave, both school and unemployment. Being single, I needed an income. After 2 years of therapy the insurance company refused to give me any extended LTD. I was still too sick to work so I had no choice but to take my pension at a reduced rate of 46%. Not a huge pension but we survive.

Hoping I was finished with sickness for food, I discovered a large lump in my abdomen. This turned out to be an incisional hernia. This time I was hospitalized for 2 nights because of all my complications.

I have been well for the last few years but now need to have my implant replaced because it is like a rock. Probably scar tissue from all the radiation.

I keep on smiling, praying, and living. I don't take any static from anyone because I have faced cancer and survived so I guess I can face just about anything. I had a lot of support, prayers and a happy disposition. One friend said I was too cantankerous to die! Life goes on and we take this gift of life and run with it.

I hope my story is of some interest because according to some of my friends I really should be dead. But it just isn't my time.

Thanks for listening

Janet Conn

Ottawa, Ontario

Breast Cancer, Stage 2

——————■——————

SMILING THROUGH

O n Friday August 18, 1995, my 52nd birthday, I woke up feeling great, we were going away for the weekend to celebrate. I rushed to the mailbox to see if there were any birthday cards. Yes one from my sister in England and a letter from the Ontario Breast Screening Clinic that I had been expecting as a result of my regular mammogram and exam ten days earlier. I opened it expecting the usual "we are happy to inform you that there were no abnormalities detected, etc."...but instead it stated that a lump had been detected in my right breast and I should see my doctor as soon as possible.

I immediately called my doctor and got an appointment for the Monday morning. He immediately sent me for an ultra-sound. He called me on the Wednesday to say that he had made an appointment with a surgeon for the following Monday.

The surgeon attempted a needle biopsy in the office but was unsuccessful, so said that he would need to do a biopsy under general anaesethic. I knew there was something serious when I got a call that afternoon at work telling me to be at the hospital the next day for the procedure. This was followed by an eight-day wait for the results (the longest week of my life). The waiting was the hardest and to make it easier I started writing down my feelings and found that this was great therapy in helping me overcome my fears. I called my diary "The Longest Week and the following seven months" – it ended up being over 20 pages long. I still read it on occasion to remind me of how lucky I am to be a survivor and how I managed to continue throughout. All I wanted was to get the results so that I knew what I was facing and what I had to do to fight it.

A colleague at work told me about a book that had helped her through Breast Cancer – Dr. Susan Love's Breast Book. It is a great book and I would advise anyone going through this disease to pick up a copy. I found that I would read a little at a time as there was so much to take in. But it did become my bible during that difficult time.

On September 6, 1995, I was informed that I had breast cancer and would require a lumpectomy. During this time, I never went to an appointment alone because there was so much information to assimilate. In fact when I received the diagnosis I did not remember what my reaction was. My husband told me that I banged my fist on the Doctor's desk and asked him what the hell he was going to do about it. I just wanted to get it fixed so that I could go on with my life.

My initial reaction was fear quickly followed by anger and even more quickly followed by "I can beat this – I will beat this". There were days when I wanted to cry – but I overcame them. Even my wonderful feline friend knew something was wrong and never left me alone. Two days later I had the operation. The next day my sense of humour took over even as the nurse was removing the dressing to change it. I was nervous because I didn't know how much of the breast I had lost and was concerned that I didn't have a nipple –in fact I joked with the nurse and asked her if I still had it before I could even look at the damage. It wasn't that bad

– 20% of the breast was removed and I still had a nipple!!! Once the operation was over, I just wanted to continue with my life and make it as normal as possible. I insisted on leaving the hospital the day after the operation so that I could attend a good friend's mortgage burning party – it was a great party!!!

Approximately three weeks after the operation, I was informed that I had stage 2 cancer and would require chemotherapy and radiation treatments. I got a call from the Regional Cancer Centre telling me I had an appointment with a Clinical Oncologist. I asked what a Clinical Oncologist did and I quickly learnt a brand new language that comes with a diagnosis of cancer. From that point on I made a list of questions and fears that I would discuss with the doctors or nurses when I went in for my appointments – this together with having my husband with me helped me as well.

My first appointment was obviously scary but the doctor, the nurses and the social workers were amazing and made me feel special and informed me of support groups and programs to help patients. The Regional Cancer Centre offered a wonderful program called "Look Good, Feel Better" – a program for women sponsored by various cosmetic companies and wig makers. There were about ten women all going through treatment, most of us bald from the chemotherapy, laughing and joking as we tried on different make-up with the help of volunteers from the cosmetic companies. We were then given products to try at home.

I know that there are many support groups for cancer patients and survivors. I myself did go to one a couple of times, but felt for me the support from my family and friends was all I needed. However, I do know that for others it is really an important part of their recovery. Everyone should decide themselves what right for them.

I decided to go back to work as soon as possible, continue my ballroom dancing lessons – this was great therapy. Usually physiotherapy on the arm is required after a lumpectomy because lymph nodes are removed from under the arm, but because of the dancing I did not require it and my surgeon was amazed at how quickly I regained motion in my arm.

I made up my mind that breast cancer was just a minor inconvenience in my life and that I would continue to do everything I had been doing before the diagnosis. A sense of humour was very important – I spent a lot of time making fun of adversity. Specifically, when I lost my hair even before the second chemotherapy treatment – my husband and I were in absolute hysterics while trying to shave off what was left of my hair. We still talk about it today. As soon as I found out that I would lose my hair because of the chemotherapy, I went out and got a wig. I was very lucky finding a lady who specialized in treating cancer patients and was very understanding and kind. I picked out a wig that practically matched my own hair colour and style. In fact once I started wearing it very few people even realized it was a wig.

Once I knew what I was fighting, I made up my mind that I might as well face it with as much of a smile as I could and work as much as I could throughout and continue my life – work, dance, time with friends – normal, everyday things. In fact, all my treatments were worked around my life.

In November 1995, after my second chemotherapy treatment, I danced at a competition in Ottawa with my instructor with my wig on. My dance instructor and I had a bit of a joke going that if the wig would fall off, we would just keep dancing. It didn't and I went on to get gold medals in all my dances.

Just before Christmas 1995, I finally finished my chemotherapy treatments and waited a month before I started a five-day a week for five weeks series of radiation treatment. Thanks to the wonderful technicians and nurses, I was able to face this with a sense of humour. Pen marks were put on my breast and under my arm where they would be doing the radiation. This quickly turned into a series of messages from my technicians to my husband and back – a heart for Valentines Day – a happy face. Once again I was laughing instead of crying.

I quickly learned how wonderful the doctors and staff at the Ottawa Regional Cancer Centre are. Their dedication and sensitivity to their patients is nothing short of incredible. They were kind, understanding and always kept a sense of humour because they know the horror a patient has at being diagnosed with cancer. From the receptionists to the Cancer Society volunteers, the technicians who took blood, the nurses in the chemo treatment room, the social workers, the wonderful staff in radiation and of course the doctors who spent as much as time necessary with me and all their patients explaining what is going on and what to expect.

In the middle of my radiation treatment, I changed jobs. A few people knew of my illness but most did not even realize that I was wearing a wig. Two weeks after starting the job, I decided the wig must go as my hair was growing back in, very short, but nonetheless real hair. The first day I had a lot of fun, from hugs and congratulations from my colleagues who knew to stunned disbelief from others and one colleague who blurted out "what did you do to your hair, take a lawn mower to it". I really enjoyed playing the role that day and never again would I complain about the wind spoiling my hair – it felt wonderful and I felt free.

The thoughtfulness and caring of my sister in England, my friends and my colleagues was paramount in helping me to face the operation, chemotherapy and radiation. They were without exception there for me throughout and it made them feel that they were contributing by supporting me. I also realized that for those few months I needed to be single-focused and self-centred in order to keep a positive attitude and a sense of humour. I also realized that my friends and family needed to support me in order for them to cope as well.

I have been cancer free since my last radiation treatment on February 28, 1996. Even though it was at times a terrifying experience, I found a lot of positives: I became spiritually much closer to my friends; I never take anything for granted; I refuse to be in the company of anyone who is negative and make a point of informing people of this. Even if this does make me a little more impatient, I don't have to listen to negative thoughts when there are so many positives and I have more self-confidence.

I went through seven months from detection of the lump to the end of my treatments and at each step I kept reminding myself that it was short-term pain for long-term gain!!!

One thing I do know is that no two patients handle a cancer diagnosis the same way nor do they necessarily have the same treatment schedule. Many people have asked me about my treatments, how I felt, etc. I tell them that they may not have the exact same treatment; treatments have changed over the years. In other words each patient is treated as an individual.

I am now 12 years cancer free and am trying to continue to live my life in a positive way. I exercise three times a week and am retired but working part-time as a tour guide sharing the wonderful capital city of Ottawa with visitors from all around the world. And yes – I am still smiling!!!

Nancy Freeman

Ottawa, Ontario

Survival ... and then some ...
from a malignant tumour of unknown origin

————————◼————————

My story is one of survival, not so much from cancer itself, as from some of the possible side effects of effective cancer treatment ... and discovering quality of life in unlikely places.

My cancer was a mystery even to the medical team. Diagnosis was difficult. Here was a patient with no family history of cancer who presented symptoms at first not able to be defined. Having lost thirty pounds after a year of decided discomfort, tests of all sorts, six months of morphine to help ease the pain, the diagnosis was finally made: a malignant tumour of unknown origin had blocked one ureter and strangled one kidney.

Surgery was decided upon to clarify the diagnosis and initiate possible treatment. The kidney was dead and was left in place. The tumour, however, the only sign of cancer in my body, defied the surgery. It was too well attached to vital organs to be removed surgically. A decision was made that, as soon as I was well enough to proceed, I would undergo an aggressive treatment of radiation.

Once diagnosed, I cannot say enough that is positive about the care I received. The care taken to reach a correct diagnosis was invaluable.

The radiation treatments proceeded well. Twenty-five sessions did the trick. My cancer has not reappeared in over five years.

However, two years after the cure, I experienced an onset of internal bleeding due to the aggressive nature of the radiation treatments. My radiation oncologist sent me to a gastroenterologist who confirmed extensive radiation damage, inoperable because burned tissue does not stitch well, and further complicated by that fact that I had internal adhesions due to several previous, non-cancerous, abdominal surgeries.

The problems: uncontrolled bleeding; recurrent blockages requiring hospitalization; one questionable kidney. The treatments: possible blood transfusions; possible colostomy surgery. The surviving kidney was struggling as well. The nephrologist team member even mentioned the word dialysis. Not happy prospects, particularly when I was feeling decidedly unwell much of the time. Guidance provided by my medical team was outstanding. The doctors and nurses made it clear to me that it was my job to be part of that team. A patient's condition will only improve if that patient does what he or she can do for him/her self. Had I not done my best for myself, I would not be writing this article today.

The bleeding: my oncologist recommended a series of Hyperbaric Oxygen treatments that are known to be effective for some burn patients. Another member of the team caring for me, my Hyperbaric Oxygen doctor, did an assessment to determine my suitability for 'immersion' in the Hyperbaric Oxygen Chamber. Deemed suitable, I was booked for forty treatments to be administered five days a week for eight weeks, two and a half hours of immersion per treatment. The principle at work here is that when body tissues receive high concentrations of oxygen under significant positive pressure conditions, new capillaries will grow, thus enabling scabbing, in effect bringing burned tissue back to a state of possible service to the host ... the host being me! Forty sessions made a remarkable difference. Not immediately, but slowly, the bleeding decreased. I felt some resurgence of energy, an element that was decidedly lacking in my life at that time with the loss of blood I was experiencing. Six months later I had an additional twenty treatments. Now I have almost no bleeding. Some foods and certain physical activities have the capability to precipitate bleeding, but that I can certainly handle!

During those many hours in the Chamber I had the privilege of getting to know several truly courageous, highly challenged, individuals. Squeaky clean, clad in antiseptic garb, not a spot of lotion allowed anywhere, hair on our heads covered, anything that might cause a spark in the highly concentrated oxygen conditions removed, two at a time we were lowered into the depths. Many of my companions were in dire straits, yet most of them remained remarkably cheerful and uncomplaining. We watched movies, breathed concentrated oxygen through our headgear, and shared many special moments that will remain with me as part of the rich tapestry of my life.

Blockages and a questionable kidney: I truly am my own prime caregiver. You, too, must do your best to take care of yourself. At seventy-five years of age I am quite capable of selecting foods that agree with my particular system. Daily doses of doctor recommended supplements keep me functioning well. Regular blood work keeps kidney function monitored. To be foolish is to risk bouts of pain, a liquids-only regimen, or more drastic treatment. To be wise is to choose to do what's best for one's self. Selfish this is not. If we do not care for ourselves, what good will we be to anyone else?

As for my cancer: regular blood work and annual abdominal CT scans inform my radiation oncologist as to my current health. I know, and am truly thankful, that he and his team are ready to act on my behalf should a need arise. We have outstanding care available throughout the Ottawa Hospital system. Every day I thank God for that!

I also thank God for my very special husband, family and friends who supported me without restraint throughout a difficult period in my life. They were all there for me in a major way, which provided much-needed strength for me to cope with the situation. Six years later I am able to enjoy those friends and family to the fullest, as well as do my part in our community to the best of my ability. What more could a seventy-five-year-old possibly hope for than that?

Zelda Shore

Ottawa, Ontario

Breast Cancer, Stage 2

———————■———————

At the time of this writing (April 2008), I am a 24 year survivor of breast cancer. In thinking about what I might be able to contribute to this project, I have had to recognize that one of the things I have done best over the years as a cancer survivor is to back burner my experience and fears and get on with living. Where the strength to do this has come from is a total mystery to me! I've come to believe that when humans need extra strength that we have it within us to draw upon – where it comes from is individual: spirituality, personality, family roots and relationships, a zest for life, a need for knowledge....I really don't know, but I found it!!!

It was May 1984. I was 41 years old, married 20 years, with 3 children ages 17, 15 and 10. I was a primary teacher prior to the birth of my children and had been a stay-at-home Mom until 1981. Having recently found very satisfying work using my teaching skills working with disadvantaged mothers and their young children, I was enjoying the balance in my life – being a wife and parent and contributing to society through part-time work. Life was good!

I must admit that taking care of myself often fell to the bottom of the list but I was diligent in doing a breast self-exam every month. Finding a hard lump on the inside/underarm of my left breast was a shock. My family physician was very responsive, saw me immediately and referred me to a surgeon. My head was spinning....this didn't happen to young women...I was still considered young wasn't I? Who was this surgeon I was being sent to....had never heard his name? I called my gynaecologist who supported the referral and encouraged me to see the surgeon as soon as possible. Again, the system worked for me...an appointment within days. A biopsy confirmed a malignant tumour. A cancellation got me a surgery date the first week of June. I fought it – the eldest children were in the middle of exams, work was busy – since this really wasn't happening, there was some mistake, waiting another few weeks wouldn't do any harm....confusion, denial, numbness were all working against me. My husband took over, surgery would happen in June. I told one girlfriend who was a constant and amazing support in the early stages and through treatment. Telling the children was very difficult...they seemed not to "get it", going on with what they were doing and leaving me feeling like they didn't care. That same evening I noticed the eldest and youngest sitting on the front steps, hip to hip. I was in an upstairs room with an open window so I could hear what they were saying – "Is Mommy going to be like Terry Fox?" I turned away as I sunk to the floor in tears...they "got it"!

You ask how does one come to terms with this disease? I'm not sure that I did. I looked at my children and I decided that they needed their Mother and their Mother needed to be in their lives, for a long time yet, so I was going to beat this disease. I was angry, terrified, went through a period of blaming myself (didn't eat properly, didn't get enough exercise, had too much stress in my life sandwiched between my teenage children and elderly parent), felt like a walking time bomb. How do you tell an aging parent that her child is potentially deathly ill?

Did I do any research on breast cancer? No. I was numb, had never dealt with the medical profession in any serious situation. I'm a more informed individual today…would likely not have made different decisions but would have done more homework had cancer struck me at this stage of my life. But at that time in my experience and I believe in society generally, doctors were not challenged or questioned. I placed my trust in the surgeon, the oncologist and in their experience. JUST GET IT OUT OF ME!!! I had a lumpectomy, 14 lymph nodes were removed and 4 were compromised. The protocol at the time was radiation therapy every day for 4 weeks followed by 6 months of chemotherapy. I don't recall being offered any treatment options and I can't even remember the names of the drugs or the regime – once every 3 weeks by injection plus 2 pills which I took daily (not sure for how long each month). My Mother was terrified – "the treatment would kill me if the disease didn't". The list of possible side effects were overwhelming…my teenage children were focussed on the fact that I would lose my hair…to me this was minor compared to other things on the list until it actually started to happen. I bought a wig, straw hats and colourful bandanas. My hairdresser, when she saw me in the wig, insisted on styling it for me….I remember joking with her to be careful how much she cut because it wouldn't grow back! It was warm wearing a wig in the summer and I was constantly nervous about if it was straight, the wind, bumping it etc, etc. More than once I threw it across the room as soon as I entered the house. Today I think I would be comfortable being bald rather than enduring a wig. I was off work all summer. By the time I returned to work I had started chemo. I fell apart in November. The weather was miserable, I had a cold which was putting my chemo off by at least a month, I was no longer the centre of attention at home, being super Mom was exhausting, some of my friends were telling me that I wasn't the same Zelda and that they liked the "old" Zelda better. A series of sessions with a social worker at the Cancer Clinic helped me to put things in perspective. Keeping my life as normal as possible was the answer for me. I arranged my chemo appointments for Thursday or Friday afternoon so I had the weekend to deal with the fatigue and nausea (Stemicil helped)....not even sure I've spelled the name of this drug correctly....it's all about putting it on the back burner!

Of-course I worry about a recurrence....in fact, more so as more years have passed. It's on my mind during those hours when I'm falling asleep or waking up....times when I'm less in control of my thoughts. How many more years can I dodge the bullet? The Cancer Clinic "fired" me after 18 years....I was taking time that sick people needed. My family physician is very attuned to my fears. She sees me regularly, is very thorough and does not make light of any perceived symptoms on my part. If I had a recurrence, would I react differently? Good question....I'm 65 not 41 but I see and desire more years ahead of me, so yes, I would probably react differently...I'd be a stronger self-advocate, I'd ask more questions, I wouldn't accept waiting for diagnosis, treatment etc. It's a different health care system today than it was in 1984....I would actively seek information, consultation and treatment. My children may be grown, but I have 2 beautiful baby grandchildren...a good reason to live longer. I say all this knowing that quality of life is also important to me, so who knows, when faced with a potential killer would I be as strong, as determined to survive again???

Support came to me in many ways – family, friends, work... as much of a familiar routine as possible. Formal support came through my oncologist, the nurses in the treatment rooms, the clinic social worker. A surprising support network developed amongst the other patients who sat in the waiting room for hours as I did. My need to engage people, share experiences, support others and laugh or cry with them stood me in good stead during those many hours in the Cancer clinic. I always had a notebook with me in which I recorded my feelings and observations. I brainstormed with myself the content of a number of proposals for work-related grants during those 6/7 months sitting in the Cancer clinic, 2 of which were funded! When my treatments were done and I had the go-ahead to travel, my husband and I went to Paris....Paris in May is lovely!

No one can tell you what you should feel at the time of diagnosis ....feelings can not be programmed or judged. My experience taught me that I was a survivor, that I had it in me to keep on going...I tire of the expression "fighting a courageous battle" but I'm not sure how else to describe that difficult year and each and every year since as I've looked ahead and moved ahead. None of us know what's around the corner, so my philosophy has been don't peak around the corner, turn that corner with strength and dignity, live life daily and BACK BURNER!

Elizabeth Keeble

Ottawa, Ontario

Breast Cancer

———————◾———————

I discovered my first cancer in January of 2001. While lying on the sofa watching television, I idly began a breast examination, something I did very sporadically. When my fingers encountered a sizeable lump in my left breast, time stopped. I remember going icy cold, totally, head to toe. I froze in position and realized that I wasn't breathing. For awhile, I was caught in disbelief, then fear and then in a complete and detailed fantasy of what was about to happen to me. I went through the surgery, the chemo, losing my hair - the whole nine yards.

I don't know how much time passed before I suddenly snapped out of it, but eventually I did. It was a Friday evening, my roommate was out and some sane part of me understood that the only person available to ground me was me. With that understanding, my practical side stepped in and I found myself calmly planning what to do next. Don't go running wildly off into a future that isn't here yet, I cautioned myself. Stay here.

Decide what the next step is and don't go any further than that. So the next day, I went to a clinic to have a doctor verify that, yes, there was a lump. On Monday I went to my doctor, who, unfortunately, was someone completely new to me. My previous doctor had left her practice and this was going to be my first meeting with her replacement. I'm sure that he hadn't expected to do anything but introduce himself to me and then book another appointment at a later date for a proper physical.

Having me present him with a breast lump must have thrown him.

Whatever the reason, we didn't get on the ball immediately, something that I find quite stunning now. I did go for an ultrasound but the results were "inconclusive". Instead of sending me for a mammogram, the doctor decided that it was simply a cyst and if I wanted, we could aspirate it.

I decided against that and left, quite unconcerned.

About 6 weeks later, it occurred to me that with this lump hanging around in there, I would never be able to tell if something else, possibly more serious, emerged in that breast. So I went back and asked to have it aspirated.

That meant being referred to a different doctor, who sent me for a mammogram. The mammogram showed a problem, so a biopsy was done. A few days later, I was told I had cancer.

Returning to my practical mode, I began gathering information about this disease. Using Susan Love's Breast Book, truly the bible for breast cancer, and the internet, I did as much research as I could handle. I spoke to informed friends and other survivors until I hit my saturation point. Then I stopped. If I couldn't absorb any more, I decided, then I didn't need anymore. I had enough information with which to make any decisions that came along.

While I was busily doing all this investigation, I had also stepped onto the cancer conveyor belt which carried me from appointment to test to appointment again. I discovered an entire sub-culture that surrounds this illness and was impressed at the compassion and support that was offered every step of the way. Every nurse or doctor or support worker I met was human and kind, a considerable feat in my opinion, considering what they are dealing with day after day.

They would answer my questions as fully as they could, direct me to other sources if they couldn't and generally met me with unfailing sympathy. I was impressed.

Concurrent with the down to earth, practical issues that I was dealing with, I was, of course, handling all the emotional kerfuffle that goes along with this diagnosis.

The first days after I got the biopsy report, I wandered around in an almost bemused state. I was having trouble taking in fully that this had actually happened to me. Me, who was slim, non smoker, light drinker and with no family history of breast cancer.

I had a good diet, eating organic whenever possible, with lots of fresh vegetables and fruit. Based on the current wisdom, I seemed a most unlikely candidate for developing cancer and yet I had. Now what?

Walking home from an appointment, about a week after I'd heard, still in my somewhat stunned state, everything changed. The cloud that had surrounded me was suddenly gone and I quite literally felt like I'd walked out of a tunnel into the light. And to explain that change, I need to back up a little.

In 1994, I became sick, more or less over night, with something that took 2 years to diagnose. While undergoing a gazillion tests to try to figure out what was wrong with me, I went on working despite overwhelming fatigue and increasing difficulties in the digestive department.

I was a ballet teacher. I had been a ballet dancer. I had spent my entire life in the ballet world. Dancers don't stop because of pain or fatigue. Our training is to carry on no matter what so the one thing I knew how to do was to keep on going despite every signal from my body that I needed to stop.

So that's what I did. I carried on until I could hardly stand. I reduced my work schedule and continued to try to push through mind numbing fatigue and crippling stomach cramps until I finally got the diagnosis of Chronic Fatigue Syndrome (CFS).

This is a very tricky and devastating illness. You look fine, but are dealing with extraordinary fatigue, sleep deprivation, sore joints, headaches, cognitive dysfunction and a host of other symptoms that make day to day living a painful uphill battle. After two years of struggle, the demands of teaching eventually became too much and I went on long term disability.

The next five years were spent fighting this disease with every fiber of my being. I spent thousands of dollars trying anything that sounded like it might produce a cure. I changed my diet, took supplements and homeopathic remedies, I did acupuncture. I saw energy healers and chiropractors, massage therapists and psychics. I was determined to not give in. I was going to get my life back, come Hell or high water.

While this was going on, my life as I had known it was steadily being dismantled. I had already lost my health, which led to the loss of my job and my income and security. My marriage went next which meant my home was also taken away. Everything that gave me my identity in the world was removed. And with that removal went my sense of worth. I had no idea who I was if I wasn't a teacher, a wife, a contributing member of society.

Three years of serious depression followed during which I maintained my sanity by continuing to do my mindfulness meditation practice, something that had been a part of my life for a number of years. This practice, along with weekly sessions with my therapist, kept my head above water.

I had been introduced, through my reading and meditation practice, to the idea that everything that comes to me is actually FOR me. That the major events in my life, happy or otherwise, are presenting themselves as gifts, as opportunities to grow and learn. That I might not like the packaging is irrelevant. My job is not to rail against what is happening but to do my best to see what the situation is trying to teach me. By approaching it with curiousity and a genuine desire to learn, I will be given something of inestimable value.

Living with CFS was the greatest challenge that I had met so far, and it took years for me to accept the obvious - I could not control what was happening. The only thing I could control was how I was reacting to what was going on. And unless I applied what I knew to be true, that there was something important to learn here, I'd never find any peace. My "take no prisoners" attitude to the world had to change.

Once that happened, all the mental and emotional anguish fell away. Although my external circumstances hadn't changed, everything was different.

So, now we return to my walking down the street, grappling with the fact that I now have cancer to contend with.

Between one step and another, I suddenly remembered all this. I recognized that cancer was no different from CFS and all that I had learned in dealing with it was directly transferable to dealing with cancer. This new situation was just another offering, another way to help me learn and grow. It was simply the next step I was meant to take on my life's path. And with that realization, as I said, everything changed.

Over the next few weeks, as I waited for my surgery, I came to believe that something quite wonderful was coming and my excitement grew. I began to see the tumour as a repository of a number of emotions and states of mind that I no longer needed. My body, in its infinite wisdom, had gathered them all together in a neat package so that they could be removed. By the time I was being rolled into the O.R., I felt lit up like a Christmas tree. I knew, without a shadow of a doubt, and for no discernible reason, that something tremendous was about to happen to me.

Throughout this whole journey I was blessed with the most extraordinary support from my community of friends. Given that we all hold a similar world view, no one met my theory that this cancer was a gift with skepticism or judgment. Instead, they embraced it along with embracing me. My wonderful roommate and I would have these inspired conversations which only deepened my conviction that something life altering was happening. And of course, they were also witnesses to the fact that that is exactly what occurred.

And to explain what did happen, I have to digress once again.

When I first moved to Ottawa, I began going out with a lovely man. We saw each other for a year and despite the fact that I knew that he was one of the "good guys", I would sometimes give him an incredibly hard time. I was critical and intolerant in ways that made me cringe even then, let alone now, but I couldn't stop myself. I meditated on it; worked on it with my therapist and even spoke with him, all to no avail.

Despite my best efforts, every so often, this anger and bitterness would erupt out of me, leaving both of us upset and dismayed.

After a year, we had to stop seeing each other. And in the following year, I got cancer, had my surgery and treatment.

Two weeks after my treatment was done, I ran into him again and we were delighted to see each other. We decided to give it another try and it was in that reconnection that I discovered the gift the cancer had brought me.

My behavior with him had completely altered. There was no anger or intolerance, just genuine caring and an open hearted communication. All the negative emotions that I'd been carrying for the last ten years, all the pain from the myriad losses I'd experienced, had finally been healed. They were gone and have never come back.

We continue to see each other. That was cancer number one.

In 2004, I found another lump and the whole process began again. There were some differences this time, however. Though the surgeon started with a lumpectomy, he came out of the surgery worried that he hadn't gotten it all. So a month later, I had a full mastectomy. The pathology report proved the surgeon right and I was very grateful that he'd followed his intuition, not to mention his considerable experience, in choosing to operate again.

The surgery was followed by chemotherapy, something I'd managed to avoid the first time, and then radiation. Having to deal with chemo created a new set of challenges and once again, my friends stepped up to the plate. They got me to the hospital and back, comforted me when my blood count was too low to allow me to use a session; they called to see how I was doing, without making me feel that I had to talk if I didn't want to; they sent little cards and emails so that I'd know they were thinking of me. But most of all, they LISTENED to me.

If I was having a hard time, they didn't tell me to be positive - really, not a doable task when you're feeling like death warmed over. They didn't offer advice or try to persuade me to be somewhere I wasn't. They would just listen, and let me know I was loved. Allowing me to be authentic with whatever was happening in the moment, whether it was joy or tears, was the most supportive gift they could have given me.

I do believe that our attitude has a powerful impact on how we walk this journey but I believe even more firmly that it is vital to walk it as truthfully and authentically as we are able. And in my experience, the most effective tool for encouraging that to happen is to stay in the moment. Stay true to what is really happening, not to what you wish was happening, or what you think someone else wishes was happening.

Recognize that no one feels up and positive all the time, and let yourself be where you actually are. When we are able to rest in the moment, without fighting or judging it, whatever is happening usually shifts pretty quickly. It's resisting it that allows it to hang on.

So, it was in that wonderfully accepting atmosphere that my friends created that I discovered what this particular cancer had to offer me. It brought me to realize that I had finally found my true home.

In the previous fifty odd years of my life, I had never felt as if I really belonged where I was. I spent most of my time feeling like I was on the outside looking in. Even when I appeared to others to be on the "inside", it was seldom my actual experience.

Now, following the second cancer, I discovered that I was a full fledged member of this circle of loving friends. There was no inside or out. There was just this circle where everyone belonged and was cared for. Me included. The recognition of this incredible connection and belonging is one of the most significant and powerful experiences of my life. I had never expected that it would happen, but it had. My heart was wide open and I knew that I was loved. As far as I was concerned, the loss of a breast was nothing in comparison to this gift.

That was cancer number two.

In March of 2008, on a now routine breast exam, it seemed to me something in my left breast wasn't quite right. There was a lot of scar tissue left over from the lumpectomy, which my oncologist and I both checked regularly. It wasn't easy identifying anything specific with all that extra tissue around but nonetheless, on this particular examination, my intuition said something had changed.

My family doctor sent me for a MRI which came back indicating that there was something "suspicious" around the scar. A mammogram and ultrasound then followed.

The scar tissue made finding anything with the ultrasound very difficult but the radiologist at the Woman's Breast Health Center didn't give up and eventually found something that seemed to stand out.

One biopsy later, which also called for patience and persistence on the part of the radiologist, and another cancer has been found.

A third diagnosis is very sobering. My first reaction has been overwhelming fatigue, truly mind numbing, bone deep weariness. I find myself face to face with my own mortality in a way that I hadn't experienced the first two times. For whatever reason, I had had no fear of dying then but meeting this illness yet again has brought it home to me that I could be in line for an earlier than anticipated death. As I said, a sobering thought and one I continue to work with.

At this writing, I've not yet had the planned mastectomy. I continue to deal with exhaustion and on occasion am totally fed up with the whole thing - I mean, enough already!! But along side these not very surprising reactions, I find that I am, once again, looking forward with some excitement to what is coming. Already I can feel a shift in my consciousness as my body and spirit prepare for the next installment of this fascinating journey. I have no doubt that something remarkable is about to happen.

If left to my own devices, I would never have agreed to living a decade with a chronic and debilitating condition followed by 3 rounds of cancer. But having survived them both I find that my overwhelming feeling is one of gratefulness for the gifts that have come to me through the medium of illness. Both the CFS and the cancer have been my gurus. They have been teachers without parallel, and even with the occasional attack of anger or fear or just plain exhaustion, I consider myself lucky to have been able to sit at their feet.

Denise Côté

Orleans, Ontario

Breast Cancer

---◼️---

I was diagnosed with breast in 1965. I was only 21 years old. My reaction was: NO, can't be, shock, disbelief, they made a mistake, impossible. I'm too young and WHY ME?

I didn't have time to build any strength. After they told me I had cancer, I was hospitalized two days later so I definitely had no time to think. They had to operate as soon as possible as the cancer was spreading really fast.

My strongest support came from my father. My mother was totally useless, she kept crying and saying nobody could take her little girl away from her. She was hysterical to the point that the hospital staff had to prevent her from visiting me because she was causing such a disturbance. I really thought I was going to die. I thought she knew something that the doctors didn't tell me.

Cancer sure did change my outlook on life. At 21 years of age, I thought I was going to live forever, that I was indestructible. Then I realized how precious life was. It was hard for me to make any kind of change in my lifestyle. I was too young. It had an awful lot of impact on my life. It was difficult when I was dating. How do you tell your date or do you even want to tell him. When is an appropriate time and how do you tell him. Nobody could help me there. I didn't know anybody that had breast cancer before. Was this a casual relationship or more? How is your date going to react? Will he leave you because you only have one breast or will he love you for who you are? I really had a hard time with that. It was always so stressing. Eventually, I did get married and had one son.

I didn't have a choice in treatment back in 1965, it was a radical mastectomy and then cobalt treatments for 3 months.

I didn't have time for research and 43 years ago there wasn't that much around, no computer, almost no literature. At 21 years of age, you really don't know too much about cancer.

I got really lucky that there were no side effects of any kind. I was told to expect to lose weight (now that was a horrible thought since before the operation I weighed 95 pounds but after the operation I weighed 65 pounds, losing my hair, getting horribly sick right after the treatments (vomiting). They even gave you a brown paper bag right after the treatment in case you were sick, and loss of appetite. While I was taking the treatments, my appetite excelled, I gained weight, never got sick, didn't lose any hair so I counted myself lucky. No side effects.

I don't worry about recurrence. After 43 years, I think I'm pretty good. This doesn't mean that I couldn't get cancer again. There's always a possibility but I don't waste my time thinking about it. I try to eat good, I walk a lot and always have a positive attitude. My father was always there for me. He gave me so much support and confidence. Every morning when I woke up, he would come into my room and ask how I was. I would tell him: Dad, I just woke up and I'm alive. I'm so happy. He would say: yes, you sure are and you're looking good and here's your cup of tea. He did that every day until I got better. Friends and relatives never wanted to confront me. They just didn't know what to say and really what can you say. It is so difficult, people tend to ignore you instead of encouraging you. As of today, I still don't know how to approach someone with cancer even though I've been there. The only thing I could say to newly diagnosed cancer patients is be strong, live one day at a time and treasure whatever time you have. We never realize how short life is and how precious life is. One step at a time, one day at a time.

Andrew Reynolds

Manotick, Ontario

Prostate Cancer

———— ▇ ————

I was diagnosed with prostate cancer in September 2001 just as I was starting a new job. The diagnosis took me completely by surprise as I had no symptoms and had just taken the PSA test after letting the requisition form sit on my desk for 6 weeks. After getting the biopsy results Gleason 7 and T3A ex-capsular prostate cancer. I knew things were serious and I would be in a fight for my life. I experienced immediate depression and had to be referred to a psychiatrist at the General Hospital. Between her strong guidance and that of my wife Lynn. I gradually came out of my funk and was able to start enjoying life again. I was put on hormones to shrink to tumor and received radiation the following summer 2002. Despite the fact that my PSA is now rising slowly which causes some concern. I remain healthy and am living a normal life and working full time. My advice to newly diagnosed patients would be to not let it become overwhelming like I did and to take it one day at a time. If you need to talk to a social worker or therapist do so sooner rather than later.

I feel that the treatment I received from Dr Malone and the staff at the General was state of the art. I was advised to not look too much at the internet etc. as that would add to my anxiety and not all of the information could be guaranteed as accurate. I attended a prostate cancer support group meeting when first diagnosed but did not find it all that informative.

I experienced the usual effects of the hormones I was on for 3 years after the radiation like hot flashes, weight gain and muscle mass reduction, but have taken them in stride considering the fact that the treatment saved my life.

Having cancer was and continues to be a life changing event and makes me appreciate living all that much more to say the least. I worry that it may come back but am thankful that the good staff at the cancer centre are monitoring me via my 6 month follow up appointments.

I certainly would be up a creek without a paddle without them.

Janet Currier

Ottawa, Ontario

Non-Hodgkin's Lymphoma

———— ■ ————

W hen diagnosed on December 23, 2001 with Non-Hodgkin's Lymphoma, I was referred to a Hematologist at the Queensway Carleton Hospital in Ottawa, and started 6 months of CHOP Chemotherapy at the Civic Hospital. Ottawa. My extended family all live in England and I felt terribly alone. Imagine my surprise when one by one they came over each month of my treatment and helped take care of me, even my brother, who had never been to Canada in all the 35 years we have lived here, came, and even vacuumed!

Friends stepped in and drove me to the hospital for treatment. My husbands' boss was sympathetic, but his work-load was tremendous and without friends and family I don't know how we would have managed.

Every day I tried to have a little treat! A cookie from the volunteers at the treatment centre, a Tim Horton's coffee, if I could manage it and a joke a day to keep me and the people around me, spirits up. I remember lying in my hospital bed and saying to the nurse how come I am bald-headed, no hair on my body, except my legs, and I still have to shave them! A head popped up in the next bed and a lady said "me too" and we both laughed!

After 6 months of treatment I felt extremely tired and kept expecting I would start having more energy. Unfortunately that did not happen. Sometimes with Non Hodgkin's Lymphoma the Chemo can actually worsen the cancer, if the timing is not right. That is what happened to me. It went from small cell to large cell.

I was referred to the General Hospital, for another type of Chemo., in November .2002, called DHAP. This time I went into hospital for 3 days to have the Chemo. Yes I went bald again. Good thing I invested in a wig! At least my hair always looked tidy and I only had to wash it every couple of weeks. 30% of people who have DHAP get kidney failure and you guessed I was one of those. So the Treatment was stopped. I spent another two weeks in the hospital recovering. It was a very scary time for everyone but the nurses and doctors were fantastic. We were becoming old friends, and they were such caring people. They always came no matter how often I called and always took time to explain what was going on. The unknown can be so frightening.

By now I had learnt to always take someone with me for these consultations. It can be very emotional and I often forgot what I had been told. If I couldn't find someone to go with me, I would write down any new information I was given and also bring a list of questions and concerns with me and write down the answers. I also learnt to speak up and ask for things to be repeated. I became my own advocate. If I felt I was not being listened to, I said so. I also learnt to look up my cancer on the Internet so I could understand the terminology and use it to make my point.

Next I was referred to the Bone Marrow Transplant Team at the General Hospital. The Bone Marrow Transplant process is a long and very involved one. It was my darkest hour before the Team decided to go ahead with it.

When at my recent check-up I asked Dr. Hupesh, "what was the percentage of people with similar cancers, who were at the same level as myself". He responded "only 40% were doing well after 5 years".

Last year I had infections twice a month and had to take antibiotics. Since then by Dr. Hupesh really listening to my concerns about my quality of life at that time, I now have antibodies intravenously each month. I am now doing extremely well. It has been a long, hard haul. I have been told I have a positive attitude and I really want to help other people cope with this disease.

Walter Stevenson

Ottawa, Ontario

Colon Cancer

———————■———————

When I was first diagnosed with cancer, although not unexpected, I felt shock and fear. Shock, because "it can't happen to me", fear mostly of the unknown, but also the fear of imminent death. I was not ready.

Family, friends, neighbours, people who I hardly even knew became instant and constant supporters. The ones I appreciated the most were those who were survivors and those currently in treatment (including a couple, both with terminal cancer).

Prior to the operation, I tried to show a positive attitude, because I didn't want to cause anyone undue worry. Privately, I was certain I was a goner. Certain to the point I left lists of where the important papers were, how much it cost annually to run the house and anything else I could think of. Then I prepared farewell letters and left them in my inside suit coat pocket. I later destroyed these without re-reading them.

Then came the big day: I went in for colon surgery on a Monday morning and was sent home Friday. Then the fun began. I was scheduled for a series of chemo treatments. It seemed that each week I found a new reaction, everything from rashes to mouth ulcers. However, when you consider the possible alternative, these were acceptable. And slowly, life became relatively normal again.

Then I noticed blood in my stool again. Back to all the tests, again: I was positive. Everyone gathered around again and was very supportive. Strangely, I was less affected mentally this time. I was hospitalized for two weeks, this time. One week was without food or water (which was administered by drip) because my stomach had been shut down. As always, the hospital staff were very professional, even managing my diabetes injection without problem. Then, daily home nursing care for some weeks. This was probably much harder on my wife and family than on me. At one point I had to move to the spare bedroom. My stomach was becoming active again. So much so that I bragged I was contributing as much gas as any car to our atmosphere. Then I began a combination of a chemo pump and radiation treatments. The major side effect of this treatment for me was anaemia.

After several more tests, I was once again pronounced cancer-free. Then the absolute worst possible occurred: my wife was diagnosed with inoperable cancer. It was in her lungs, bones, liver and ovaries. She was given chemo and radiation to try to slow the disease down. Even tried a "new discovery – last chance" treatment. The one decent part about this was that with the assistance of daily home nursing, we were able to keep her at home and in familiar surroundings until the last day.

Life slowly came back to what passes for normal. Then, bingo! Guess who has colon cancer – again. This time I had a colostomy and am currently wearing a stoma appliance. I can only say that it is not as big a problem as I first pictured it. It even has a couple of advantages which I will not go into here.

The above narrative has taken place over a period of five years. I am now 77 years old. It is not an experience to be treasured. I do consider myself most fortunate in having the best medical expertise and caring home nursing to help me recover. And front and foremost has been my family, who are always there.

Elta Watt

Arnprior, Ontario

Breast Cancer

———————■———————

W hen I got diagnosed with breast cancer, I felt sadness, fear, concern, upset, overwhelmed, alone, end of life. Then I got mad and decided to fight this thing that came into my life to rob me of a future. My husband and family were the strongest support for me.

My lifestyle changed. I learned to appreciate each day and every petal on every flower was so beautiful. I learned that material things were meaningless and life was very precious. I also made many changes in my life, my faith grew and God was always first and foremost in my life. I cast all my fears and unimportant things away. I know from the moment I was told of my diagnosis that I had no control over my life. I was sitting in the palm of God's hand and everything was of his will.

The impacts on my life were very strong. I had to do what I felt was needed to get me over this interruption on my journey in life and be there for others who needed my help. We go through life not knowing what tomorrow holds, but we need to be open, ready to accept the unknown, realizing that our lives are in God's hands and we are here to love others, care for others, support others, and just be there when you are needed. Seek out people who have been through this journey and ride along with them.

I felt very good about the medical advice. When I was getting the advice it was like hearing a foreign language spoken to me. I had no previous knowledge of medical treatment for breast cancer. I felt that the people I was dealing with were the experts and I needed to trust their decision.

When my treatment was set up I did get very involved in the research of my diagnosis. People, books and internet were a great source of research for me. There were no support groups around our community. I tried without success to find some, feeling very alone, having no others on the journey to talk to. So I decided to start a support group which has become the largest active support group in Ontario. When I started the support group I said if I could help one woman it would be of great benefit. Today our group has helped hundreds of women who have been so distressed at receiving their diagnosis.

As for side effects, I felt blessed that I did not have many. There were two things that affected me: one was being claustrophobic when they put my shield on and bolted me to the radiation table, and the second was losing my hair (being a hairdresser). I took a "positive" attitude towards being sick. I would constantly nibble on light things such as crackers, plain toast, puddings and yogurt. I was determined to beat this nasty thing that has crept into my body and tried to end my life.

At the beginning I did worry about recurrence, coming up to every appointment I was a nervous wreck, I would get myself so worked up. Then one day I realized that I had no control over the situation and I needed to live every day, enjoy each day and love each day. I keep very busy, I try to keep fit and healthy, I don't worry about things that I can't change and in general, I just love life.

I am very blessed that I have not had a recurrence but I deal with people every day who have gone through a second diagnosis.

I stand at awe at them, they are so strong with a wonderful spirit, a strong belief and determined to kill the beast once again.

When you are well known in a small town and change your hairstyle to a wig, people catch on (saying that she must have cancer), but I always tried to dress it up a bit.

My suggestion to relatives, friends and co-workers on how to interact with newly diagnosed cancer patients is to be there for them. Cancer is not contagious, listen to them, be a shoulder for them to cry on, hold their hands, hug them, and show compassion.

Ten months after I was diagnosed with breast cancer, my husband had a heart attack so the focus shifted quickly from my recovering from surgery, chemo and radiation treatments to his health concerns. I had to be strong for the two of us. I had gone from a recovering position to caregiver. Then a few years later, we lost our first son to heart disease. It has not been easy but through it all I hold on to my faith.

A year after I had my diagnosis, I went for a doctor's appointment and the news was good. When we came home I went to our bedroom to change. My eyes seem to be drawn to the window only to see the shape of an angel on the glass. I will never forget the feeling I had, it was just like God giving me confirmation that everything was going to be alright. I knew that I was about to embark on a new journey, a journey that would have me helping others. Here I am 15 years later celebrating the wonderful journey. I have met so many beautiful people along the way; my new friends became my family.

I have inherited a short verse from the Italian/Spanish culture which I live by each day, I would like to share it with you "Vota Vita Mia" meaning I dedicate my life.

My message to all of you: Believe, Pray, Love & Hope.

Blessings & Love go out to all of you.

Dan Alexander MORRISON

Ottawa, Ontario

Colon and Rectal Cancer

———————■———————

I write this in 2008, 43 years after my first encounter with cancer. I have had three recurrences since, each one being dealt with successfully by having surgery. I would like this account of my survival to give a hopeful message to others in a similar circumstance. Having cancer doesn't have to be 'the End of the World' for a person.

In 1965, after three years in England, teaching Chemistry at a Grammar School in London, I decided it was time to go back home to New Zealand. I answered an advertisement for a teaching position in Canada, and decided to emigrate to there. In August, I crossed the Atlantic in the Queen Mary, arrived in New York carrying in two hands everything I owned, and ended up at the Lambton County Collegiate and Vocational Institute in Petrolia, near Sarnia, Ontario. I shared accommodation with another young man and started teaching Grade 12 chemistry. Near the end of the school year, I started to experience digestion problems and could feel a lump in my upper right abdomen, which turned out to be in the transverse colon of the large bowel. The doctor ordered X-rays, which had to be done twice, because he couldn't believe that someone at my young age (29) could have a tumour. I would say that my initial reaction to the diagnosis was philosophical; I felt rather helpless, knowing that there was nothing I could do to change anything, and was resigned to letting things take their course. I went for surgery to the Sarnia General Hospital, and had a colonic resection. After I spent 10 days in the intensive care unit, the surgeon had to operate again to deal with adhesions. Before leaving the hospital, the surgeon talked with me saying I shouldn't let this episode get me down, to continue my life course, to make plans, get married, etc. I had already decided that having a Master of Science degree, teaching at high school was not for me, so I applied for a teaching position at community colleges in Ottawa and in Windsor. At that time teachers were so much in demand that I was accepted by both, by telephone.

I was fortunate that a colleague kindly let me convalesce at his home for a week or two. I had already purchased a 1954 Dodge Station Wagon (for $100), so I then started a three week 'camping' trip through southern Ontario, on my way to Ottawa, visiting holiday locations (such as Wasaga Beach), and sleeping in the Wagon. On arrival, I checked in at the Ottawa YMCA, and reported to the Eastern Ontario Institute of Technology (at 200 Lees Ave), where I was given my work load, which was mainly to teach Physical Chemistry to 3rd year Chemical Technology students.

I perused the 'Shared Accommodation' ads in the newspaper and ended up sharing a house with two other guys, about my age. At that time, the YMCA had square dance lessons, so I joined the 'Dip'n Dive' club, as my way of adopting a bit of North American culture. It was while 'dipping and diving' that I met a Swiss woman, who was there for the same reason, and we were married in 1968.

I had been referred to an Ottawa specialist, and had regular check-ups. In 1972, I noticed I was passing some blood, and it was found that I had malignant rectal polyps. The surgery which followed, in September of that year, removed my rectum and created a colostomy, making me impotent. Fortunately, I already had a baby son, born the previous February. The new colostomy, with the appropriate appliances, belts, etc took some getting used to, but I managed. The main concerns were the problems of smelling bad, and how to change pouches. In those days, few of the appliance systems were odour-proof, or even air-tight, or secure. I soon investigated and adopted the technique of irrigation, which involved introducing water into the large bowel, in order to clear it out. By this means I was able to go two days without an appliance, use one on the third day, and irrigate again on the fourth. This technique was fairly common in the UK, but not so in the USA. In 1978, I was granted a sabbatical leave, and spent a year in Suva, Fiji at the University of the South Pacific's Institute of Natural Resources, analyzing water samples from inland and around the coast. Social events and trips were organized by the 'Fiji Rucksack Club' consisting mainly of 'ex-pats' from other parts of the British Commonwealth. Being able to participate with these others was reassuring for me to accept that I was in fact back in the 'land of the living'. By then I had mastered managing my ostomy, and experienced no problems with air travel, or with the tropical climate. Back in Ottawa in 1979, I started having what would be politely called 'digestive problems', but were in fact cramping pains in the large bowel, due to peristalsic action passing fecal matter through the large intestine. X-rays showed that I had a tumour in the ascending (right) colon. So at the Riverside Hospital, for my third cancerous encounter, I had another colonic resection. Although the surgeon said I would no longer be able to irrigate, afterwards I did manage to do it every second day.

Over the years, appliance systems evolved and slowly improved. Although all were now odour-proof, the biggest concern remained, appliance failure, leakage, and smelling bad. I received the most helpful guidance and advice from the Ottawa Chapter of the United Ostomy Association (based in the USA), and I regularly attended its events and Board meetings. The Ostomy Association of Canada has since split off, and the local group is now called the United Ostomy Support Group. In 1981 we hosted, and as President of that group, I organized the first ever bilingual Annual Ostomy 'Capital Care/Soins Capitaux' Conference for the Central Northeast Region of North America.

I would say that I reacted philosophically to these occurrences, taking them in my stride, knowing that whatever fate throws at you, one could and should make the best of it. I remember, the night before surgery, lying in bed and thinking that if I live through this, to the best of my ability, I would devote my time and talents to making the world a better place for those less fortunate than I.

Resuming work at Algonquin College, I taught a reduced timetable of three days per week, for ten years, finally taking early retirement in 1996. In the mean time I had joined and become active in many volunteer groups, including the Unitarian Church. I had a bad road accident in 1992, giving me a head injury and a broken back which gives me constant pain and discomfort to this day, adding to the drawbacks I have to deal with.

Because it was time to make a visit back home, I flew to New Zealand to attend a 1998 'cousins reunion', and to spend some time with my mother. It was the last time I saw her because she died in 2005 aged 91. My father had previously died of stomach cancer in 1941, when I was only 5 years old. Adding to my burdens and struggles, my dear wife left me in 2001. I say to people that living alone and without companionship is a bad enough fate, worse even than being a cancer survivor.

In 2007, I started having cramping abdominal pains, similar to what I had experienced before, especially during peristalsis, and with a tender spot at the left end of my transverse colon. A colonoscopy and biopsy confirmed a malignant tumour. The surgeon said that there was so little colon left, that it would all have to come out. So after a total colectomy, I was left with an ileostomy. The good news is there is now no odour problem, but instead there is a major concern to avoid leakage and skin excoriation. As well, having to change the pouch at least three times per day, has put limits on my activities. The other good news is that in none of the four cases was follow-up radiation or chemotherapy necessary. Each instance was unrelated, with no metastasis, and having the surgery was a complete cure. I put this down to early detection, and diagnosis. I am now being monitored, just in case, by having three-month CTscans.

My advice to others is to learn, recognize, and not to ignore any unusual symptoms. Annual visits to a family doctor are not enough; one must be aware constantly of one's own body, and take the initiative in cases of doubt. In my case, no doctor ever detected symptoms before I did myself. Doing nothing or hoping it will go away, is not only foolhardy, but verging on suicidal. Many cancers if caught early enough are survivable, and can be successfully dealt with. As it is said in another context, but is vital in this:

'Time is of the essence'.

Bryan Tyrer

Ottawa, Ontario

"Collision" tumours: andocarcinoma and endocrine carcinoma

———■———

A pparently, I am a very rare case indeed. I had what they call «collision» tumours: two different types of cancer in the same spot. There have been only 32 cases reported, world-wide, since the early 70's, of this anomaly occurring.

The 1st cancer is: glandular, relatively slow developing and, because it was detected in a very early stage, pretty much contained in a 4 - 5 cm. tumour; this is a lesser concern. The 2nd cancer is endocrine carcinoma with andicar carcinoma cells, hormonal, very rare in its own right (doctors at the General are aware of only one other case), very aggressive, fast growing and terminal; obviously of greater concern. I have a 5% chance of surviving this one, or at least surviving for a few years. By default, I have a 95% chance of not lasting much longer. On the one hand, the surgeons are quite pleased and confident that they were able to remove all the cancer they found. This entailed cutting out a good portion of my esophagus and a part of my stomach where the two meet. Because the cancer had gone through my stomach wall, they also removed all the lymph nodes around my stomach and pancreas, the one of which contained cancer cells. I don't really have a stomach anymore as it was stretched into a tube to resection my esophagus ... now, whatever I eat goes straight to the small intestine without any place to be digested. This does cause some issues but nothing that I can't handle.

Normally, the 1st cancer would be treated with some follow-up, precautionary radiation, but because of the location there is a significant risk of permanently damaging healthy organs like the kidneys and pancreas, so the doctors are recommending against it. With the 2nd cancer, there is very little historical data. None of the specialists can say whether chemotherapy would have any effect or not, and this treatment is very debilitating and invasive; the side effects include nausea and vomiting, joint pain, loss of balance, difficulty walking, hair loss, loss of hearing, low white blood cells, bruising and bleeding, mouth sores, bleeding gums, seizures, etc, and just for good measure, it attacks all the cells, good and bad, and destroys the immune system which means you are at great risk of infections, viruses, etc, so the cure can kill you.

So, given that the specialists have no idea whether chemo can help, and given that they have no idea regarding timeframe (a year or two - ten or twenty years - likely the former but who knows) with or without chemotherapy, I have opted to not go through the treatment. I'll take that 5% chance for now, quality over quantity. I'm feeling pretty good right now, back into some light work-outs with the weights and some other physical activity. My wife Connie retires in June and we have a lot of things we want to do together and places to see (back to Graceland, visit places like San Antonio, Tombstone, Italy, Barbados, etc. and of course, get a Harley Davidson". So, I'd like to enjoy what I have rather than take questionable treatment with no guarantee of any advantage and be sick for months at a time. I'm making up my «bucket list» as we speak. If/when the cancer shows up again, I may revisit my decision.

Connie and I met with the doctors on Monday and it turns out to be a sort of «good news/bad news» kind of situation. As I have mentioned, I have the very rare distinction of having 2 different types of cancer in the same area. This sort of complicates things. The chemo I'm getting is intended to target the very aggressive, fast growing and more dangerous of the 2, and appears to be working in that some of the cancer is shrinking, but the other cancer is growing. To illustrate, let's say I have 10 spots or areas of cancer that show up on the scans (the doctors can't tell what type is which on the images); 6 are shrinking and 4 are growing, including the redevelopment of the cancer in my throat/esophagus that was initially removed through surgery.

We go to Plan B: although they can't do radiation on my abdomen because the cancer is in my kidneys, liver and pancreas and radiation would permanently damage these organs, they can do radiation on my throat; another round of CT Scans to benchmark and I start radiation. In the interim, they are trying to get me into a «clinical trial» situation (have to qualify and be accepted by the team of specialists) in which some experimental drugs/ chemotherapy, that have been successful in attacking a variety of types of cancers, would be used; waiting for news on that front.

In the meantime, my last round of chemo had to be postponed (2nd time) as my white cell count/neutrolites was too low and thus the risk of totally wiping out the immune system and leaving me open to fatal infections etc. is too high; this is the part where the cure could kill you before the cancer gets you. I am up to my ass in appointments, tests, scans, chemo, radiation; don't know what I did with my time before all this.

Plan C, if needed, would involve a PICC (peripherally inserted central catheter) inserted in my upper arm or chest (Morgan Freeman had one in The Bucket List); this eliminates the need to insert IV's for the chemo 20 or 30 times a session and allows for virtually 24/7 chemo treatment on an out-patient basis. The chemicals also come in pill form but they would cost $2,000 every 3 weeks and, of course, are not covered by OHIP.

The confusing part is that I feel fine, physically and otherwise, doing all the things I want to do, no real side effects, pain, sickness or discomfort, even my hair is growing back in. It's sometimes hard to comprehend that something really bad is going on inside.

I had a PICC line (peripheraly inserted central catheter) put in. It's like a mini-operation, local aesthetic: an I.V. needle is permanently inserted into the upper arm and then a catheter run through a vein in the arm, up over the shoulder and into my chest just above the heart. The upside is that I don't have to be poked and jabbed a dozen times whenever I go in for treatment. I was getting concerned that if I ever got dizzy and fell down in the street I would wake up in a rehab lock-down because of all the needle tracks on my arms. Now, with the PICC line they can use it to put stuff in (chemo) or take stuff out (blood samples) without reinventing the wheel each time. I have to keep it covered and dry and a Home Care Nurse sees me once a week to check my vitals and change the dressing. The downside is that the PICC means they feel it is necessary to step up the programme. It also allows for 24/7 chemotherapy. I did 5 days of radiation on my throat last week.

The radiation treatments were quite efficient. I had a card with my appointment schedule, other basic information, an identification number and a bar code. Each day when I arrived, I could check the computer screen for my identification number and be informed as to whether things were on time or delayed, and by how much, for the specific radiation machine that was assigned to me. Then I scanned the bar code and the computer automatically registered me in, let the radiologists know that I had arrived for my appointment and slotted me into the waiting list. No human contact.

Once I got called in, usually pretty much on time, the treatment only took about 15 minutes: line me up on the bed thingy, check according to my tatoos (yes, I have permanent tattoos, just little dots to line me up properly each time. Thankfully it didn't involve a butterfly on my aging butt), then calibrate the machine and ZAP.

During the initial consultation, I was asked if I used any facial or body creams and was advised not to during radiation treatments. Most creams have metal in them and it would be like wrapping something in tin foil and putting it in the microwave.

When I finished the radiation and had a CT scan, I met with the surgeons and the oncologist. I'm assuming that we'll get a status report and some inkling of whether anything is working and where we go now.

Apparently, when the team of cancer specialists get together for the weekly case review, I'm the hot topic of discussion, such a rare bird that I am, at least I know they're paying attention; surprise, surprise, they don't always agree. This past week, I met with the 3 of them for a status report and I think, it's generally a «good news» scenario, or as good as might be expected, all things considered.

Dr. Seeley, the surgeon, wants to do a barium scan. The CT scans only show what's on the outside of my organs and gastrointestinal system; the barium scan will show what's on the inside, particularly in my throat area. If I continue to have difficulty swallowing, one option would be to stretch out my oesophagus. A second option would be to insert a permanent stent; not thrilled about this one. It would mean I would be on a soft food/mush diet for the rest of my life (you can't imagine how often I dream of a big BBQ steak). Life is just one irony after another. There is my little granddaughter, Sadie, being introduced to semi-solid/soft foods, and here is her grandpa possibly being introduced to semi-solid/soft foods and we both have the same hair and wrinkles, although I think she might have an edge on the former and I have it on the latter; what goes around comes around, life is really just one big (or small) loop and you pretty much end up where you started. The process would be pretty much a colossal waste of time if you don't do something of significance or value in the time you have.

Dr. Chow, the oncologist, is a bit of a pessimist, only reluctantly offers any good news, but very efficient and informative. The last CT scan indicates (not withstanding the re-emergence of the cancer in my throat) that the cancer appears to be now confined to my liver and some surrounding lymph nodes and has not grown (maybe even shrunk a bit) since the previous scan. I think that's pretty good news but Dr. Chow wants it to be better than that.

She did say «Don't get the stent!».

She is still trying to get me into the Clinical Trial programme. There is a spot right now but I'm #3 on the list, she's trying to see if she can «leapfrog» me into the programme because of my special situation (collision tumours/2 types of cancer etc The trial is sponsored by Pfizer and using a couple of experimental drugs (probably a combination of oral/pills and 24/7 drip through my PICC line). The drugs are approved by Health Canada and the U.S. Food and Drug for clinical use, sort of the step between testing on animals to using on humans. I am not sure exactly where I fit on the spectrum, maybe the «missing link» between the two.

Dr. Grimard, the radiologist, is quite confident that the radiation will address the cancer in my throat but it will take a few weeks to realize the effects. Funny, I just assumed that the radiation would be instantaneous, sort of like Captain Kirk's laser; ZAP! OK you're cured. Apparently, depending upon the type of cancer, it could be anywhere from 2 to 8 weeks before you see results. He said I would know in a week or so just by my ability to swallow; if it doesn't improve then we'll do another round.

I did the Barium test to see about the difficulty swallowing; what a nasty little process that is. Fast for 12 hours then the first thing you get to eat is about a gallon of the Barium stuff, stand on a little platform in front of a screen (the technician can move it back and forth sort of like one of those ducks in a shooting gallery and he can move the X-Ray scanner up, down and sideways), take a big mouthful of Barium, hold, swallow, scan; do that about 10 times, then knock back a cup of some kind of crystals (I think to create air/gas in the upper GI - gastrointenstinal), wash that down with a slug of Barium and start the whole process again. After that, I don't care how long you've been fasting or how hungry you might've been you really don't feel like eating. Don't have results yet but a follow-up appointment with the surgeon.

I couldn't get into the Pfizer Clinical Trial/Study; 3rd on the list, an opening only every month or so, due for my next round of chemo but have to be off 4 weeks before starting a new programme, etc. The timing was off and the pieces weren't fitting, so they got me into another Clinical Trial/Study sponsored by Bristol Meyers Squibb. Apparently, only 40 people from Europe, U.S. and Canada are accepted, and I am number 6 here and feel so special.

Once again, I went through a lot of tests, prerequisites for approval and benchmarking, Echogram, ECG, PET Scan (no I'm not being treated by a Vet) and lots of blood work. I swear that I am under the loving care of the Transylvania Medical Team, their appetite for blood is voracious.

The PET Scan involved another 12 hour fast, then they inject a radioactive isotope dye through an I.V., lie down for an hour while it circulates and settles in, then on your back, arms over your head and stay perfectly still for an hour while they run you through the scan, arms/shoulders getting sore, cramping up, an itch on my nose. I don't understand why the Ontario government doesn't support or encourage PET scans, virtually every major hospital has a machine, it can detect small cell cancer that CT scans can't so, presumably, earlier detection and treatment, maybe a better chance of survival, but most people have to go to Québec or the U.S. at $2500 a pop; I don't understand.

In the Clinical Trial programme on day one I get prepped (vital signs and, yup, more blood work) then 6 hours of chemo (paclitaxel and carboplatin); did this last Friday. I got a new anti-nausea prescription specific to these chemicals but I couldn't find a drugstore that had it in stock; had to order it and go the weekend without medication, not good. The team was shocked to find out on Monday.

On days 4 through 19 I take the trial drug (pill form) BMS-690514. On the 1st day of the pill, I spent the whole day at the General to be monitored over 8 hours, more prep work and, yup, more blood work. I got the pill at 9:17 a.m. so I have to take it at exactly the same time every day (control purposes, I guess) but I have to fast 4 hours before taking the pill and 3 hours after, so I get my 1st coffee and something to eat around 12:30. The 1st day, they took vital signs every ½ hour, blood work every hour and an ECG every 4 hours, final physical and finally got to go home. After 21 days, I get a couple days rest and then start the whole cycle again, possibly for months or years.

In between I have to do more blood work and monitor my blood pressure on medication as this is one of the side effects.

You really have to wonder sometimes; they really want me to gain some weight but I have to fast for 8 to 12 hours each day of the trial. The pill is the size of a football (maybe not quite) but one of the side effects is difficulty in swallowing. The test drug causes diahrrea but the anti-nausea medication is constipating; maybe I'll get lucky and just break even.

Anyway, that's where I'm at right now; pretty tired and not feeling great but, hanging in.

Brigitte Davidson

Ottawa, Ontario

Breast Cancer

I was diagnosed at 29 years old after finding my lump 10 months earlier.

At 29 in 1995 it was difficult having a physician take a breast growth seriously. I was easily convinced that shouldn't worry about it as I was too busy planning my upcoming wedding. The day I went to get my marriage license was the day that forever changed my life. I met up with a childhood friend at the license bureau and explained to her that I all was great except for this annoying lump that kept growing. She then urged me to have a biopsy as her cousin had passed away recently at 36 years old due to an undiagnosed breast tumor.

That night I went home and cried uncontrollably knowing deep down that I had a long struggle ahead of me. Somehow I always knew. After my wedding, I insisted on a biopsy. The news came December 23rd, 1995, 9 weeks after being married, I had to tell my husband and family I too had breast cancer. My sister-in-law was diagnosed in 1992 and was now in terminal stages of breast cancer making it very difficult for my husband and family to cope with yet another sickness in the family.

Having no benefits, as both my husband and I had just started new careers and had not yet qualified for a drug plan, you could only imagine how I was more worried about making ends meet than making it through this illness.

Somehow we made it through.

I wished to reach my five year anniversary. Somehow that magic number would unlock my fears. Within one week of my five year anniversary, I conceived a child. He is now 6 years old and life continues.

June Humphries

Ottawa, Ontario

Colon Cancer

—————————■—————————

I always tried to be physically fit with participation in organized and individual sports (although to a lesser amount in my 40s when I changed careers), had never smoked and maintained a reasonable diet (NOT perfect, and certainly not meeting "Canada Food Guidelines" for fibre, vegetables and fruit). I was never seriously ill during my working years and only hospitalized once (appendicitis). Life was great! And longevity is a factor on both sides of my family history.

Did I suspect cancer when I went to my family doctor for tiredness, several weak spells that caused me to leave work and get drives home, some indigestion below the chest bone and an increasing inability to climb stairs without stopping, especially at Lees transit station when I returned from work? NO. These symptoms are indicative of a health problem for several major and minor diseases. I was not overly concerned but recognized that something was not right within my physical body. I believe that one must tune in to the rhythms of their body and be aware when it reacts.

The tests began. Waiting times can seem endless, but the progressive pattern of my tests moved swiftly from initial complaints (November) to diagnosis (March). Two ultrasounds and a barium enema were negative. Finally, a blood test revealed I was anaemic (not always listed on the colon cancer symptoms list) and my haemoglobin level continued to fall in spite of mega doses of iron. Thanks to the persistence of my family doctor, I was finally diagnosed after several endoscopic tests, the last one being a colonoscopy.

When the gastroenterologist saw me before I left the endoscopic unit, he told me I had a cancerous tumour in the ascending colon (right side) and surgery would be required. I felt like I was on the receiving end of a cold, matter-of-fact, clinical statement that lacked empathy for me as a person. I was in shock and shed a few tears because I had heard the dreaded word "cancer". Initially, my response, like many others, was "but that's a man's disease". As a single woman, I had learned to be independent in the work world and to make and trust my own decisions. Without much thought, I told him to make arrangements for surgery appointments.

The surgeon made me feel at ease, let me see the photo of what I termed "that little sucker that's causing my problem", explained the process, and even called me at home the night before surgery. This unexpected thoughtfulness of a caring professional relieved some of my tension, especially when we joked about the "cleansing solution". He seemed to sense that I was putting on a brave front, making my own decisions and yet feeling alone and afraid. Easter had just passed and perhaps my later humour in the operating room helped me as I joked about "the last person tied down with arms outstretched like this was nearly 2,000 years ago". Humour is a definite asset with any disease diagnosis.

Next stop was the Cancer Centre. Fully expecting to be told I didn't need any treatment because surgery had gone well, I again was shocked by the assessment that chemotherapy was required with two options - standard 5FU and leucovorin or a clinical trial. Trusting myself, I opted for the tried and proven for my Stage III

(T3N0M0). I reacted to the first set of treatments, but with dosage adjustments further reactions were almost non-existent. During treatment, I received strong support from the oncologists, my family doctor, a social worker, Community Care Access, Meals on Wheels, and several co-workers. I almost quit the chemotherapy after three months because I hated those dosage needles, but my family doctor and the social worker were a strong factor in my decision to continue. My family (brother, sister and sister-in-law) verbally supported me. My brother was critically ill during my last several months of treatment and this added to my stress; he died one week after I finished chemotherapy.

About two years after diagnosis, I decided to attend a general support group "Healthy Connections" for any type of cancer. Although no one had colon cancer, their stories and problems were an incentive to me. In my third year, I was part of a group of interested individuals who met and formed the Ottawa Support Group for Colorectal Cancer patients, family and friends. I have learned a lot from the shared experiences. Support groups provide valuable experiential information in a secure climate. They helped me but they are not everyone's "cup of tea".

Through my gastroenterologist who forwarded my name to the Ontario Family Colon Cancer Registry, I have participated in their province-wide project. What I learned about my family was fascinating - more cancer on my mother's side; heart on my father's side; siblings - three out of four with cancer (deceased younger brother (kidney/bone), me (colorectal), older sister (breast); father - metastasized cancer; aunts, uncles (eight out of 15 mother's side), cousins - various cancers. Through this Registry, raw data is available for other studies on nutrition, exercise, genetics, etc. in relation to colon cancer.

Five years of follow-up by an oncologist and testing helped to build my confidence that cancer can be beaten. I am nine years a survivor. I still have a hidden fear that cancer will return in another form, but I maintain a positive attitude. My recommendations - remain positive; have a sense of humour; eat nutritiously; maintain a fitness level; find support (family, friends, co-workers, family doctor or support group); and **believe cancer can be beaten**.

Ray Desjardins

Ottawa, Ontario

Colorectal cancer

―――――――■―――――――

It was December 1994 and I had just completed 35 years of Public Service (13 ½ years abroad in the US and the UK). The Government of Canada was in the process of reducing the size of its workforce and offering premiums to anyone who would consider retiring early; after all I was just a young lad of 54. The offer was exciting, the premiums enticing; and there I was on January 5th 1995 retired and the future looked extremely bright. After 3 decades of tourism marketing experience, my services as a Consultant were in demand. Just great, the gods had finally come together and my wife and I were looking forward to the "Golden Years", all that travelling etc.

In the late spring of 1996, I started having minor problems – no serious symptoms of any kind, but things just didn't seem right with my digestive system; and despite working with my GP, we couldn't find anything. Then came the crisis and I was referred to a specialist on an URGENT BASIS. My wife and I visited the doctor together and she waited in his office while he examined me. He took my history and a biopsy right there in his examination room, told me to dress and return to my wife in his office. When I returned, there on his desk was the vial with the piece of material he had removed and he had also placed a full body chart beside his desk. He then very carefully explained that what he had found was a 'raging' tumour in the rectum that he was certain was cancerous.

It was very close to my body with only 2mm of clearance and that 15mm was the normal separation required surgically to ensure a positive result. I had colorectal cancer and it had to be removed as soon as possible. Using the body chart he showed us that my colon would have to be diverted to create a permanent colostomy on the left side of my body. The prognosis was unsure and would depend on how successful the surgery was. He ordered a series of tests, arranged a visit to a haematologist to ensure I could give 2 pints of blood for use during the operation and bumped another of his patients so I could be operated on October 24th 1996. A very thorough plan of action.

As my wife and I were paying very close attention to what the doctor was saying, we didn't react until he had finished. We turned, looked at each other in stunned disbelief - realizing for the first time that my life was on the line. WHY ME? We walked back to our car in stunned silence, which I can only describe as a "pregnant pause"! What could I say, my life flashed before me with a sense of overwhelming despair! Is that it? - all I had worked for, all we were going to do – it's over – I'm a dead man. How could it happen to me? What had I ever done to deserve this? It was a very quiet long ride home that afternoon. I was frightened, anxious and totally consumed by the diagnosis, what had to be done, and my mortality.

Later, after the initial shock wore off, I began to realize that I was not alone - my wife, my children, my brothers and sisters and their children, my church brothers and sisters, and friends began to rally around me. I could talk, I could cry, and I did a lot of soul searching of my life story to date, and the thought that my life could end in the very near future. This made me deal with the future - for my wife and children, the preparation of my Will and Personal Powers of Attorney.

I began to think of each day as if it could be my last – so I lived it to the fullest. The things I had collected, owned, etc. suddenly were no longer of value. Most importantly, I reconnected with my spiritual beliefs as a Christian and began to look in the Bible for all the positive statements relative to death and what was to come. I re-read the passage about the "laying on of hands" for believers, those who are ill and I asked my Pastor if he and the Elders of my church would perform the ceremony. I found this a very key moment in my attitude changing, from one of hopelessness and helplessness to one of real hope as I realized I was not alone; there was a Big C on my side!

On Thanksgiving weekend, all my siblings and their families joined us for our Thanksgiving Meal. After the meal, we all gathered in the living room and we talked. I heard myself reassuring them that all was well whatever outcome (frankly as I think back, I can hardly believe the strength I had gained.) Before people left that day, my sister-in-law who was in training as an Anglican Priest and my brother who was a Minister both lead separate "laying on of hands" family ceremonies. I was truly surrounded by love and I felt it both emotionally and spiritually. This seemed to be a very important event and turning point as I began to deal with coping with the realities of my diagnosis, the possible outcomes, and how I was to begin really looking after me.

Since the surgeon had been very frank and informative, also mentioning that survival would probably include "impotence", I was determined to find out all about the type of cancer I had and the fact that if the operation was successful, I could end up being an ostomate and probably impotent. So I began the collection of brochures from the waiting room at the Civic Hospital and books and flyers from their library. The more I learned the more I wanted to know and this lead me to a meeting with the Chief of Surgery and his assistant who were in the process of a large study on family genetics and its relationship to colorectal cancer. This resulted in the donation of the material that was to be removed from my body so it could be used as part of their research. I will return to this later, especially its relationship to my own family history and what resulted for my siblings and my children. The critical point is that all this "busyness" and curiosity kept my mind off the surgery and began to increase my level of hope that there was a strong chance of survival. Then came Oct. 24/96 – 5½ hours of surgery and waking up in the Recovery Room just as they were giving me back the last of the 2 pints of my own blood. Yes I woke up – I was alive, I had a colostomy bag on and my lower body had been altered but I sensed that things had gone OK. I was on the surgical floor a few hours later.

It was 2 days later that my surgeon came in and sat at the end of my bed. He had come to share the report from pathology. For the 1st time in nearly 6 weeks, I believe I saw a slight, very slight smile on his face. He had done a very "radical" surgery but had removed the tumour; he had also taken 7 slices of lymph node from the area all around the tumour, destroying a massive number of nerve endings. However, the pathology report indicated that all slices of lymph node were cancer free. I was cancer free, and his recommendation was some follow-up radiation after I had fully recovered from surgery and was healthy enough. What a relief, so much so that I can't remember what I felt. However, I did have the presence of mind from the additional reading information I had picked up to ask him if he would also refer me to an oncologist-chemotherapy – which he did. With the new life I had just been granted, you can imagine the effect on my rate of healing – I was home on the morning of the 7th day after surgery.

It was an initial three month healing process because of the extent of the surgery. Because my wife was at home recovering from a smashed knee (resulting from an accident almost two weeks before), my daughter-in-law stopped her home business and became our principal caregiver. After my recovery from surgery, I was given two weeks of chemotherapy and six weeks of radiation. It bowled me over for another three months. In fact I am still looking for the license plate number of the 18 wheeler that hit me. This was a total of six months of weakness, deep depression, and constant nursing. During the first three month period, the "busyness" I had developed before surgery now became a large part of my coping mechanism from two aspects – understanding what was going on and my support groups. My contact with the Chief of Surgery first came into play. As a result of the colorectal study we created, a Family History which indicated that I was the third generation of males on my mother's side to have the disease (illness in families were never spoken about in the past.) So contact was made with all my siblings to have a colonoscopy immediately because they were at risk genetically. My son and daughter were also tested even though they were only 36 and 39. Everyone was clean except my son who had a benign polyp removed. My children are now on a 3 year follow-up routine. It turned out that when my material was tested, it was a "new" gene that had mutated and only partially. This resulted in further research by the Loeb Institute to determine if for some reason this particular gene had been missed in their earlier work.

Helping others is a great way of helping yourself! During the final three months where the weakness, depression, and overall hurt was most pronounced yet again one of the things I had discovered during my information search period paid great dividends. I had found that the United Ostomy Association - Ottawa Support Group existed and had a Hotline that you could call. This Hotline became my lifeline as I could call and talk to other ostimates who had gone through the same thing I had and were willing to listen, share their experience and provide all kinds of advice to deal with my colostomy. This was particularly critical during the period I received Radiation as I suffered considerably with burned skin, a very debilitating problem for a new ostimate. The sharing and caring of a Support Group I cannot overstate.

Having someone to talk to, who has experienced what you are going through, reinforces the fact that you are not alone, that what you're feeling is normal and that your health and strength will return. This group extends to your family, friends, and all those with whom you are involved. It's tough to share, to cry, to let yourself say and feel what is happening to you with others. It's hard to be so vulnerable but in my experience, it's a life saver. Talk, talk, talk, and read and read and learn about what's going on. I can assure you that it will lead you to a new life of wanting to help others, to belong to service clubs and groups in your community so you can give back just a little of what you have received. In my case, I became a Certified Hospital Visitor for Ostomy patients, a Hotline responder, and a member of the Royal Canadian Legion, a Director on a number of Boards dealing with Youth, Community and Veterans' issues. Sometimes it pays to be busy to minimize your own health issues while continuing to understand that there are so many who have much greater burdens to bear and needs even you can help meet.

Do I think much about the possibility of a return of my cancer? The obvious answer is, of course. However, I have developed a lifestyle to deal with my busyness – eat healthy, keep active and deal directly with the limitations of a colostomy – both in terms of what I can eat, when, so it does not disrupt my schedule, simply accept that I will have mishaps and be prepared for them and learn to live with the memories of those things I can no longer experience in life. Sounds onerous but its amazing what you and your body can adjust to, what you can do without and how much you can achieve.

I have already had a return of another form of cancer "basal cell" so I am very careful to respond to any lumps or bumps. With the wealth of data I have now read and collected and my ostomy training – my safeguard is my action rather than reaction. I am always conscious of anything unusual as I know they can be significant. I also visit my doctor on a monthly basis and have an annual check-up including specific tests related to my cancer and those that men are most susceptible to, to keep informed and react immediately. Don't expect anyone but you to be responsible for your health.

Don't buy into fear – cancer is being beaten everyday. Your best safeguard is to react and attack your symptoms immediately. It has always been the best defence.

MICHAEL

Glendora, CA

Non-Hodgkin's lymphoma

———————■———————

Living with any serious disease can be a test. If you or a loved one has been there, perhaps you can identify with my story. We all hear the mind-numbing statistics: one in four people will have some form of cancer in a lifetime; one in three families will see a loved one live, perhaps die with cancer. (**Source**: *American Cancer Society*)

Still, such data seems sterile and unlikely, until the day cancer hits home.

For me, cancer came home when I contracted one of the most aggressive forms of non-Hodgkin's lymphoma (NHL) in March 2006. The day began like every other workday. Rising to shower and shave, I discovered a lump under my right arm, a growth about the size of a golf ball, also about as hard. What's this? I finished showering and getting ready for work while contemplating: What now? This was only days before my wife Dee Dee and I planned to begin a Florida trip to visit family and attend my 40th high school reunion (the first I have attended since graduation). Because there was no pain from the site of the lump, I decided to wait until our trip was over to check the matter with my doctor (and my wife).

Upon returning to our California home a week later, another week passed before my doctor's appointment. Still silent with my wife about the discovery, I returned home that Thursday evening, finally sharing that I had seen the doctor that day about a mystery growth under my arm. Astonished that I had been so stoic and silent about the matter, Dee Dee, quizzed me for answers I did not have and wouldn't have for some time. I was glib. She was puzzled.

The next step was a scheduled appointment with a thoracic surgeon for a biopsy. By now, we were certain this was not just an infection because other growths had appeared. When the biopsy was completed and diagnosis confirmed, the cancer reality was ours to live: mantle cell lymphoma (MCL - aggressive blastoid type).

This is a chapter of our lives still being written over time. The book is incomplete. Initially, we had an HMO referral to an oncology group that just did not connect with us in the proper way. Our second referral was much better and that is where our treatment began in April 2006. Originally, the oncologist scheduled eight sessions of chemotherapy. After six sessions, I was in remission. He advised me to call his office in six months to schedule an appointment to develop a maintenance plan. Unfortunately, ten weeks later the cancer returned. When we were referred at that time to another specialist (thanks to our point of service (POS) option in our HMO plan), we began a third cycle that started to employ some weekend inpatient treatment in addition to the continuing outpatient therapy. By then (and we knew this was likely to happen), referral came to a major national cancer treatment center in the area to start the therapy that would lead to the stem cell transplant. Because we never obtained lasting remission from some 16 different chemo treatments, our only viable option that offered hope of a cure for MCL was a stem cell transplant. The unrelated donor stem cell transplant (MUD SCT) was completed on August 22, 2007. On the 44th day post transplant, results of a PET scan were negative (cancer gone!) and we also received the DNA test results -- the SCT was successful. My blood type, DNA, and immune system had been transformed to that of my 23-year-old anonymous donor somewhere in an overseas location. Presidential hopeful Barack Obama tells of weird and unexpected genetic connections in his heritage. My stem experience attests to the homogeny of the world's gene pool. My own two brothers were not matches. A total stranger was.

Looking back over my two-year survivorship to date, I remember one day, when we arrived at the hospital outpatient clinic for a chemotherapy appointment, the registration line was particularly long (maybe 50 people). Falling in line behind me was a middle-age woman with her husband and from her first comment I overheard, I could tell that this was their first visit. She remarked: "Look at all these people; how sad!" I couldn't help but respond to her: "This is not sad at all. All of these people have this place to come for care, treatment and a possible cure! What would they do without this hospital?"

Just prior to our stem cell transplant procedure and hospitalization, our physician and medical care team informed us that we had a 10%, possibly 20% chance of success with this treatment. This evaluation largely came from the fact that the lymphoma was so aggressive. Since the beginning of chemotherapy (April 2006), the longest period of remission had been ten weeks (after the first treatment). We found that most of the succeeding treatments would bring shorter-term remissions; some none at all. The greatest risk complication from the stem cell transplant procedure was graft versus host disease (GVHD) which can be fatal.

Meanwhile, until Nov. 30, 2007, I was restricted to home confinement for the first 100 days of recovery. Nearly 250 days post-transplant to date, recovery has been steady but slow with some skin rash (GVH), but on Feb. 25, 2008, I returned to work on a part-time basis. The partner and wife that I was so reluctant to share those first signs of the disease (because of some silly male trait that tries to foolishly protect loved ones from harm and bad news), has been my most constant support. She has tended to every possible need that I have had while still keeping her composure and outward strength. She was and is my best supporter and advocate. I know this has been a real struggle for her; often difficult. But she has persevered in an amazing way. Undaunted she is because of her faith and the confidence that we, together, witnessed in the care, knowledge, skills and service of our many care givers, our loving family, and a strong community of faith.

In the mind of every cancer survivor is the question: What if cancer returns? Knowing that life affords no guarantees, there is no element of surprise here, but possibly disappointment. We have survived one round; we know this is a marathon, not a sprint. We can survive others, although there is virtually no likelihood a second stem cell transplant would be done.

Research continues on the discovery of a lymphoma vaccine and perhaps that will be available in the near future. We have been asked about lessons learned during this cancer journey. The question prompts us to share: If possible, we would not, in the future, take a course that would have us see so many specialists on our way to the best care destination we could have found. To those who are fortunate enough to have employment-based health insurance: look seriously at the point of service option (POS), if available. This affords the most flexibility and peace of mind when care providers may need to be changed. For the rest of our life, we hope to stay in the care of the physicians and hospital where we had the stem cell transplant performed. This is one of the best, if not the best, cancer treatment facilities in the world: City of Hope in Duarte, California.

Today, I am an unabashed advocate for this life-saving facility; also for the imperative that we all should keep no secrets and live each day to share with family, loved ones and friends the best that faith and hope can offer. Building such values in others is a certain way to fortify same in ourselves. My cancer story has led me to adopt: "Consider what's important, not just what's urgent." But then, of course, that is no improvement upon the classic Rotary consideration: First, is it the truth?

Dona Fitzpatrick

Ottawa, Ontario

Inflammatory Breast Cancer

———■———

I can't say I'm a breast cancer survivor yet - but I can say that I'm surviving happily and able to look at each day as a new beginning. Although the cancer keeps progressing and my doctor has diagnosed it as "incurable", I'm still optimistic that we'll manage to get the cancer completely under control or we'll find a cure somehow. There's wonderful research being done and new cancer cures being discovered every day. It's what keeps me hopeful.

In brief - I was diagnosed with Inflammatory Breast Cancer (IBC) 3-1/2 years ago. IBC is the most aggressive form of breast cancer and the prognosis was really not good several years ago. It still isn't wonderful, but there have been tremendous developments in the past 10 years or so. I feel quite impassioned about helping raise awareness about IBC and have given many public talks. Early diagnosis is crucial. The symptoms are a slight rash on the breast, or a wrinkling of the skin, like an orange peel. Very often IBC is misdiagnosed by a woman's family doctor and she's given an ineffective treatment for several months. The delay can be deadly - IBC is so aggressive that every day counts. When I was first diagnosed, my husband and I read information and statistics about it on the Internet and were terrified. Survival beyond 5 years was almost unheard of. Must admit I cried that night. Since then there have been wonderful advances with the disease and I've spoken to others who have been IBC survivors for 12 years now – and still counting.

Fortunately for me, the medical care I've received has been amazing. I have 3 wonderful, supportive and caring doctors who work as a team to help me. Days after my surgeon saw me and told me I had IBC, I started on chemo. I then had a mastectomy on my left breast and then radiation. At that point (10 months later) it looked like I was cancer free. The cancer came back in October, shortly after I had agreed to be the spokesperson for Ottawa's Run for the Cure. I stood in front of everyone on Parliament Hill that year and promised to come back as a "survivor", not just someone surviving cancer.

Since then I've had at least 8 other rounds of chemo. The cancer has spread to my skin, the chest wall and around my lung - and this year I found another primary IBC on my other breast. Last February I had another masectomy. The chemo sometimes stops the cancer growing, but then the cancer cells learn to adapt to the chemo drug and it becomes ineffective. I'm currently paying about $1,600 every month for my chemo drugs. There's a drug on the market called Avastin, that has had wonderful results in the U.S. with IBC patients. Unfortunately, it isn't covered for IBC patients in Ontario and is very expensive.

But I'm still optimistic . I've tried every natural therapy I can think of to support my treatment, including a macrobiotic diet. Perhaps the natural treatments are having an effect and working to prevent the cancer from progressing more, I'm not really sure.

Throughout all the treatment and chemo, I've managed to work full-time. I love my job and the people at the office have been wonderfully supportive - some even joining my team, "Dona's Divas" for the Run for the Cure this year. I still do everything

I used to do, just a tiny bit slower (and I have to get to bed early and get lots of sleep). Other than that, I have absolutely nothing to complain about and a ton to be grateful for. I can't believe how wonderfully supportive family and friends have been - I feel surrounded by love. People talk about the lessons they learn from having something like cancer. I feel it has taught me a lot of life's lessons and I'm a calmer, happier and more balanced person now than I ever was before. I'm grateful for every day.

And I know I will join the ranks of the "survivors" one of these days.

Mary Mongrain

Ottawa, Ontario

Breast Cancer,
Stage II ductal carcinoma

———————■———————

Journey into the jaws of cancer

After showering you rub and dry and check out the wet spots and then oops, a strange anomaly on my left breast. Just left and slightly lower than the nipple was a dimple, not one of those beautifying facial Shirley Temple dimples. This dimple was in the wrong place. Because I had a medical background (R.N.) I recognized it immediately. I had cancer. There was a big decision to make, and every time the news media reminded me to make it snappy.

In 1986 my husband was diagnosed with inoperable lung cancer. That is when the tectonic plates under the earth's crust collide and shake you up as never before. I looked after him at home for eight months. On June 17th his 74th birthday and father's day were combined and all the family came.

A week later he died as I held his hand....

So why was I hesitating? Was I hoping my end would be as peaceful as his?

It was February and I made my plans. First of all I wanted to go to Vancouver where I had previously lived, see my son and daughter who were still on the west coast, and there were my friends. I spent a couple of weeks in March there, not telling anyone of my suspicions. .I felt more or less okay, the hills in Vancouver always made my legs sore, and I accepted being tired from all the running around. When I got back to Ottawa, I followed my usual routines. I was suffering terrible pain from an infected tooth which subsequently had to have a root canal, and capped.

I have osteoarthritis and osteoporosis. The sciatica nerve was being pinched into a horrendous crippling pain. .And it was April and my 86th birthday was coming up and no way was I going to tell my family (I have five children, the two out west, two in Ottawa, and one in Wales) about my suspicions until after we had our birthday party.

So why did I postpone this for so long?

Denial? How can you deny something that is so certain. Well I really didn't deny it to myself, and as long as I didn't tell anybody I wouldn't be forced to face up to the facts and do something. I dreaded the reactions and the feelings I would have to inflict on those whom I loved most. To every ear that hears the word cancer, they also hear death. I didn't want to hurt anybody. Not too bright, right! One part of my silly brain kept thinking why not just let it go? The knowledgeable part of the brain reminded me there was no guarantee that the lump would stay quiet and just slowly kill me. It could and would metastasize It could and just might burst inside the breast. So stop being such a devout coward. And do something.

I made an appointment with my family doctor on Thursday, April 27. When he took a look he immediately made an appointment with a surgeon for Monday, May 1st.

I live in Centertown, Ottawa, conveniently close to my doctor, grocery shopping, and close to the bus. The designated surgeon had his office in the West End, a very long bus ride. He took a biopsy, and a week later called, he had gotten a false negative result.

On May 10th I went back for another biopsy.

On May 15th a call came from the surgeon 4 pm. Can you be here by five? No, no, but of course I will be. Waiting for a bus at rush hour, masses of bodies, breathing in the nauseating exhaust and fumes from the long line up of the commuter buses in unseasonably hot and muggy weather was not pleasant, to say the least, followed by a bumpy ride in and out of the potholes of Carling Ave. Finally, 5:30 p.m., surgeon's office not quite empty, but hushed, the stillness filled with foreboding. Yes it's malignant, booked for surgery June 2nd at Queensway Carleton, again further yet to me psychologically and geographically at the end of my world. Appointments at the Merrivale lab, another long two bus rides away, a mammogram, and ultra-sound, bone scan, including the roof of my mouth, they were thorough, no wait, efficient, professional and gentle.

Then, the appointment at the Queensway Carleton Hospital for pre-op assessment at noon on May 18th. I have a card to use para-transpo, the public transportation for the elderly and handicapped, but anyone who has tried to book the day before the ride is needed, has a very narrow window of contact only after 9 a.m. By the time you dial and redial because of the busy signal they're all booked. So I took a cab; thirty bucks and twenty minutes later, I arrive at 11 a.m., an hour early. That was okay, I didn't have long to wait. Everyone was very efficient and pleasant; very encouraging and complimentary on my spryness. "For my age".

First there was the nurse with the usual questions for a case history, informs me I'm booked for day surgery. I insisted the doctor had told me I would be in probably two days. She would check and let me know. (Informed next day I could stay overnight.) The anaesthesiologist was next who asked me questions of my medical history. He would not be the one administering the anaesthetic, he just made more notes. Then another doctor who asked my history, lifted my blouse to have me take a deep breath, and poked the stethoscope around my upper chest. She made more notes. Then came the lab, blood work, chest x-ray, etc.; waited a long time to be called to the physio department, then waited for the physiotherapist who when she finally arrived went through the book, warning me of the dire consequences if I didn't engage in the exercise regime from day one after surgery. Finally, the social worker came to arrange for a visiting nurse to look after the drainage and dressings at home. They all added their notes.

Decided to take the bus home, it was a big mistake, long hot and dirty ride, I arrived home 6 p.m.

On June 2nd accompanied by two sons and a daughter, I arrived at hospital at 9:30 am. I am in OR by 11 a.m. it seemed old and not quite as bright as I remembered an OR, to be.

So as is my usual wont I start blabbing away, when suddenly I feel someone give me a good shake and a disembodied voice said: it's all over. I must have been hit by a hammer, went into a deep blackout and now groggy and still trying to take everything in I was staring at the moving ceiling as I was being pushed down the hall. I had chosen to stay overnight in a ward, four in a room. Save two hundred dollars. .My children are standing at the foot of the bed, uneasy as any one could imagine, with smiles and words of support when I'm served a meal , macaroni and cheese and cold canned peas. I think they must have snickered when they saw my hospital dinner plate. Remembering the teasing they always give me about serving them cold peas. The stories so often told and retold that ties the family into the unit. What goes around comes around?

That night I spent in the snake pit, the vomiting, the effect of the drugs, the hallucinating and the neighbouring patient crying all night: "to cut it off, take it off, I don't want it, cut it off" referring to her I.V. that had been cuffed and taped to prevent her from tearing it loose.

The nurses were so calm and gentle, efficient and professional, the generals on the front line.

When my family arrived the next morning I was ready to leave. They couldn't reach the surgeon, so I signed myself out. I had arranged to spend two weeks in an assisted living place, and I was so relieved to arrive at the residence .to convalesce: Definition: from the Latin valescere 'grow strong' .to gradually recover one's health after an illness or medical treatment...I was hoping the Romans in their Latin language had said it right.

It was only one month from May 1st when I first saw the surgeon, to the day of surgery June 2nd. After all the horror stories of waiting list I thought that was quite good.

I hadn't yet begun to realize what was in store for me.

It was time for the visits to the oncologists. I was accompanied by one of my sons, Dr. Verma, well-known in research at the Ottawa Cancer Clinic gave us the statistics for survival.

Well there was no way I wanted chemotherapy and he agreed it might be a bit much. So we decided on the tamoxifen the specific drug for breast cancer.

Next came the radiation specialist, Dr. Meng whose patience with me would wear thin with my hemming and hawing and my never-ending excuse to avoid radiation, I'm too old. My tumor was less than 2 cm in greatest dimension.

I had a lumpectomy and removal of axillary nodes, a very clean surgery, and a scar tissue indentation in my armpit. I should worry about wearing a sleeveless dress? I don't think so.

So Dr. Meng went on to encourage me

She said chronologically you are in your eighties but biologically in good shape. Okay.

I agreed to 25 treatments, five days a week, five weeks.

Every Thursday I would get a schedule for my treatments for the following week. Because the time was not the same every day I could not book the para-transpo. However, the cancer clinic could arrange with volunteer drivers to pick me up and bring me back home after the treatment. This was very special because these drivers were all either survivors, or had been touched by someone very close having been diagnosed and treated. There was an exchange of stories without divulging anything personal. For instance, one whose wife had had T-cells treatment for a brain tumor. I had no idea we were so far advanced. There was a genuine kindness and empathy creating a bond between any and all who had either personally or had a family member agonize over the terror of the disease.

When a driver from the cancer clinic wasn't available I turned to the senior's community center, "The Good Companion". The cancer clinic charged nothing, the center charged twelve dollars for pick-up and return, again a wonderful contribution to morale. And there were always friends and family. I was truly fortunate in having available so much help.

Before the radiation treatment started I had to go in and be "measured" for the precise position for the rays to do their job. So I have a permanent dot (I called it my invisible tattoo) in the center of my chest, quite invisible.

The waiting period for the radiation was longer than I had hoped. The surgery was in June the radiation began on October 12th. This wait was considered borderline really. However, as they say, let the treatments begin.

In the civic hospital was the receptionist desk, where you received an electronic card that you would insert into the designated slot and whoever monitored the patients would know you had arrived. The dressing or undressing room and into the non-elegant blue not- for-dancing gown, then the wait for your turn. You were led into a huge room, no windows, probably lead-lined, furnished with that threatening single slab, dead center of the room.

Not too uncomfortable. Two technicians now took over placing me in a correct position... I listened as they called out the co-ordinates which I presumed had to be precise, and which I had carefully stored in my memory bank, in case they made a mistake.

The surgical sight exposed, with left arm curved around my head and then they all left, they went down a short hall and turned a corner where they sat behind an impermeable glass window (bullet proof maybe?) Where they had the buttons to work and by remote control, this terrifying robotic chunk of metal reminding me of the *Canada arm* used to do work in space, on its hinges moving ever closer to hang over me, ready to do its repairs, with no visible human to handle it as it swung into position to zap, here and then a whirr and a zap there, and I can't remember how many zaps, but I did not dare move a muscle, an eye lid, not because I was physically restrained, but because I willed this monster to target the spot...that only spot. It didn't take long in real time, there was absolutely no sensation of invasive treatment from the monstrous machine.

"That's it Mary" a disembodied voice freed me to relax.

Twenty-five treatments! Every day, sometimes early in the morning, sometimes later, but never daring to miss one. As it progressed, the skin darkened and burnt, but I think maybe because I'm olive-skinned, or I'm just like a politician, thick-skinned, the burning was tolerable and soothed with the application of an all natural cream called candula. The first few weeks I was not feeling too different than usual but then as the treatments continued these waves of undescribable fatigue would grip me, not forcing me to bed, with an illness, but enticing me to stop, lie down, rest..rest.

There followed the prescribed follow-ups with both oncologists. Since breast cancer cells have a tendency to metastasise into the bones, I had another bone scan, which at that time proved negative. Now it was just a matter of getting on with it, my affairs in order and back to as much living as I could squeeze into every day.

When I left the doctor's office after my first visit with my son, I had said to him: Steven, (and I repeated the same to all of them)

I am 86 years old, I have had a long and good and eventful life, sometimes, extraordinary, as you all have known. It seems who ever designed the universe said *to all things there is a season, a time to live and a time to die.* So be it now or later, as much as I might want to kick and scream against the inevitable, it's there and I will be ready."

Every day during my treatment for Cancer, I sat in the waiting room looking around me at the people coming and going, young, middle aged and old, all there for the same reason: to receive radiation, chemotherapy. My heart ached for the young women who had been diagnosed, came to get their treatment then took off to go back to either work, young families, or whatever their life entailed.

I asked myself how many of these people would be here if they had to pay for the thousands of dollars for treatments that insurance premiums might not totally cover. A personal example: young woman in the State of Washington had a tumour on her uterus. What was her choice? I can't go to see about it, I have no insurance she said.

I feel that I received excellent and timely care, for which I was profoundly grateful But for convalescing, I was fortunate enough to go to an assisted living residence. I was also fortunate to have the same daily visiting nurse to look after the drainage the dressing and assess my progress.

Universal health care is our Canadian icon: the newest cutting edge of medicine available to everyone.

The system will send in a health care giver to help with personal hygiene, and if lucky you might get one that will do a bit extra, but it is not in the job description. The community centers offer help and services for a reasonable rate. The meals on wheels will cost you five dollars a day. Para-transpo will transport you to your appointments (when you can get one), for the cost of regular bus fare. Sounds pretty good. But you have just come home from the hospital maybe the same day or after an overnight stay, or even a couple of days. This is after surgery, surgery where the surgeon invades your body with a scalpel to remove the offending cells.

The after effects of the anaesthetic can be horrendous. The drugs for pain will put you in a stupor. The effort of just getting out of bed will sometimes be too much. The consequences, if documented, would show repeat visits to emergency or re-admission, and/or severe complications. And even in the assisted living place, you are expected to get dressed and encouraged if not directly pushed to go to the dining room, where in pain and discomfort you sit and are expected to socialize.

How many patients understand what their doctors ask and procedures explained. And in the case of the woman who had been told by her doctor to go to the emergency to have an urgent blood test done. She had the blood taken, was told to wait and ten hours later she is still waiting. Maybe you or I might have started screaming, but there are people who put themselves into the hands of the professionals with total trust.

Some kind of advocacy should be made available at least for the most vulnerable to accompany the person, just as an interpreter is required for a foreign-speaking person.

And people must learn to take responsibility for their choices, for their behaviour, for their lifestyle and care for their own bodies.

Pouring money into the system is good if it doesn't disappear as it has for years, in a bottomless well of waste, inefficient workers, and the high salaries of too many administrators.

No point in buying new high tech machines if there is nobody around who can run them, not only for a few hours a day, but constantly, 24 hours a day, seven days a week, until the backlogs are cleared. If doctors are not being paid enough, come to some reasonable compromise.

Then there are the nurses. Wake up people, the nurses are your front line. They are the ones there to observe, to administer, to follow through. And when a patient wakes in the night, sick and scared and he/she pushes the call button, the nurse is probably dealing with several other tasks, but she'll be there, with the kidney basin to vomit in, an injection for pain, a dressing to cover the wound.

Is my judgment prejudiced? Of course. But if you have ever been in hospital you know it is the unadulterated truth and without exaggeration.

I was a registered nurse studied at the University of Ottawa School of Nursing in the dark ages of depression and war, and no national health system. When the wards were thirty patients lined up in four rows in a large room and there were no miracle drugs, until sulfa came along, and no technology except for X-rays, and the crude beginning of nuclear medicine in the shape of radium pellets carried around by the radiologist in a lead lined suitcase he carried as far from his body as his long arms could extend.

After graduation I did district nursing in an outport in Newfoundland which was still a British Colony and the people on the dole lived on six cents a day and whatever fish they could get out of the sea. There were still fish then. But the poor diet and living conditions caused up to 80% or more of the people to be infected with tuberculosis. I delivered babies in hovels, without running water and electricity.

The one and only doctor left in that vast and desolate area began the first universal health care. He asked the people to pay a few cents monthly, whatever they could afford to cover all their health needs.

After the war, the working people usually through their salaries paid for health insurance to a private company. After having a baby, women remained in hospital at least seven days, sometimes ten. Surgeries required at least ten days. This kept a person quite debilitated and increased the danger of embolism, and/or pneumonia. I am not sure of the life expectancy but one was considered old at fifty, and when one was sixty or seventy, they were very old. The mentally ill or physically handicapped were relegated to institutions, where they might sit listlessly hours on end. So who would want to go back to those miserable times? Not I.

We now have these multi-million dollar machines that spit out the precise details of the conditions of every organ, every inch of the human body. The pharmaceutical book is now larger than any telephone book of the largest city in the world. And if all the doom and gloom portrayed by the nay sayers against modern medicine could answer why are people living longer with better quality of life than could have been previously expected.

I am grateful and appreciate all the medical care I received in the past two years. Yes, I am a two year survivor. The cohesive group of the doctors, nurses, technicians, the kitchen staff, the cleaners, the receptionists, the messengers, each important in his/her role.

Old friends and the new friends giving their time and effort!

There is a final encompassing contribution to my well-being, It is the sharing of the teasing, the laughing, the crying, the memories, the sadness and joy, the problems resolved, the loyalty, not only to me, but to each other, the embracing palpable unconditional love of my family.

Richard Patten

Ottawa, Ontario.

Non-Hodgkin's Lymphoma

———————■———————

In August of 2000, I had come home from a cycle and a little workout and as I often do, I checked my pulse. As I did, I felt this lump on the side of my neck and I thought, "oh my God." I had lost a brother 30 years ago to Hodgkin's cancer and I recalled that he had had a lump on the lymph gland on his neck and he subsequently died at the tender age of 27. Hodgkin's disease today, if you had a choice between what I had and what he had, you would choose what he had. Mario Lemieux survived Hodgkin's disease and today it is very treatable and the chances of success are very high.

I arranged a meeting with my family physician and he said, "You should go to a specialist." He referred me to an Ear, Nose, and Throat Specialist, and he said, "Well you know, sometimes these lumps are inflammations. Maybe we should get an ultrasound" and I said, "Fine." That took several weeks. The doctor's office informed me that the doctor would see me in five weeks. I said, "Five weeks? If I have what I think I have, that is a lot of time. I think I would like to see him earlier" and she said to me, "If the doctor thought it was that serious, he would see you tomorrow."

So she was doing her own diagnosis, I suppose. So when the diagnosis came through, I hope she reflected upon what she had said to me.

Now 3-1/2 months had passed since I first discovered the lump and the review of the ultrasound. Then finally he said "Maybe we should go in there and take a look at what is there."

I had the results of the biopsy, November 9th when I went in to see the doctor. I had a wee bit of anxiety, as you can well imagine and I saw by his serious facial expression that the news was not good. He said, "We have a challenge before us, and indeed, you do have Lymphoma B Non-Hodgkin's cancer." I was hoping for better, but all right, I said, "Well how long have I got?" And he said, "This is not a death sentence." He said, "We are going to refer you to the Ottawa Regional Cancer Centre and you can begin treatments immediately. They are having very good success with this kind of cancer." I was stunned. I remember driving from the doctor's office back to my office thinking, "How am I going to explain this? I don't want Penny my wife and my family or my staff to feel upset, but of course, it was a very difficult time because you are not sure if you are saying goodbye and you are not sure what the future holds. I immediately got onto a computer and I thought "I better look up what all of this is about". I am not sure which one it was, but it was either the American or Canadian Cancer Society and I found Lymphoma B-cell Non-Hodgkin's and the first thing it said was, "Six to 18 months untreated." So I thought, "Boy, I'm in trouble." So then I went on to the next page and it said, "But if treated, 50/50." I said, "Okay, 50/50 that's fair enough, I'll take those odds." Then I read, "If it is diagnosed early, then the success rate is 60% to 70%" and I said, "Okay, hopefully, it was diagnosed early." So I thought, "I have got to be strong, I have got to learn fast, and I have got to do everything that I can do to fight this and I have got to learn as much as I can about this cancer."

Several weeks later, at my first meeting with the oncologist, the doctor suggested that I have 6 or 8 bouts of chemo over 6 months, a cocktail of drugs which would kill any cancer cells that might be floating around in my body. I would start a whole series of tests, including many blood tests and a bone marrow test and he said he would try and get me a CT scan. He said, "Hopefully," which meant he wasn't sure whether he could arrange one soon. This was at the Regional Cancer Centre beside the General site of the Ottawa Hospital. I had worked at CHEO as President of the Children's Hospital of Eastern Ontario's Foundation (1990-95) and we had actually raised money for a CT scan for the Children's Hospital. The staff at CHEO offered to do my CT scan and agreed that they wouldn't charge their time and they would give it to me free. I was concerned that I might be bumping someone else from the waiting list. The President of CHEO said, "You got the CT Scan machine for CHEO so we are happy to help you. Besides, we do not use our machine full time so you actually make room for someone else on the adult waiting list at the Ottawa Hospital."

I ran into a number of friends in the native community and I must tell you that as a particular single group, other than friends and family, the native community was the most responsive and helpful to me. I met a young woman who was a native from New York State whose name is Ann. She now lives in Ottawa. I met her through a friend of mine who said "You should sit down and talk with Ann." And I said, "Fine, I will do that." I sat down with her and she just looked at me for awhile and she said, "You know, you don't have cancer anymore. You did, but you have a very sad soul" and she said, "you have to work on your spirit." So I said, "Okay, I would do that." She was right. I was discouraged and depressed with Politics at the time. I was an MPP in opposition.

One day I got a phone call from Bill Shilling, an elder from the Rama Reserve near Orillia, Ontario, whose younger brother Arthur was a very famous aboriginal artist, and he said, "I read in the Toronto Star that you are sick." I said, "Yeah, I have cancer." He said, "Have you heard of ESSIAC?" I said, "Yes, as a matter of fact, I am using it now." It is kind of a concoction of different herbal medicines that are put together. He said, "How many ingredients are in there?" and I said, "There are three." So he said, "Well, there are actually eight. We didn't give away the full recipe because every time we give away our medicines to the white society, we never get anything in return. We don't get a red cent (If you will pardon the pun)." He said, "I am going to get the medicine man to put this together and I will get you a six-month supply and we will send it to you." So I said, "Bill, you know that is great, thank you. Look, I want to make sure I pay for this." "No," he said, "There is no way, you can pay for this." I said, "What do you mean, I can't pay for this?" He said, "We are not allowed." I said, "What do you mean you are not allowed?" He said "When we have a friend who is sick and we have medicine to address that illness, we are not allowed to take anything in exchange." What a wonderful social concept, their own OHIP.

Why did I take Essiac in the first place? Well I had read about it and there was some general success with it by a number of people, most was anecdotal information.

At that time I hadn't received the results of my chemo. I had spoken to the doctor and he said I should have a series of tests including a CT scan. I had to wait for a few hours after the scan I had taken at CHEO and while I was waiting, I was talking to two doctors I used to work with (Simon Davidson and Peter McLean), outside the CHEO coffee shop when the Radiologist came by with the results and she said, "Here is your negative. Everything is just fine." I was so happy, so much so that I burst out crying because I was so relieved. It is amazing to realize sometimes how much built up emotion you have related to important expectations. So, friends and colleagues, family, all kinds of people came forward with suggestions, with ideas. At one point, it became overwhelming. I tried everything that sounded promising. I would spend hours trying to figure out what I could take and what I could not take with what. I was spending a lot of money on numerous potions, herbs and vitamins and I thought "this is too much, I had better simplify this. I saw naturopaths, nutritionists, dieticians, herbalists, and I found that the

naturopaths were very helpful. Again, it was a woman w
me go through an audit of myself spiritually and ment
physically and otherwise, attitudinally, which I found very he
and also to look at a variety of things that help strengthen th
immune system. Most of what I learned was outside of the regular
medical system. The relationship with my first oncologist I found
worrisome because it felt like I was going in to see a technician,
get treatment, leave, and that's it. The staff were under tremendous
pressure, making it difficult for them to give you time.

From December 2000 to May 2001, I had chemo once every
three weeks and by the time I got all my tests together, all my tests
were negative. There wasn't one positive test. The only positive
test was from the biopsy for the tumor itself which I found very
interesting. As the tests came in, the doctor said, "You never
know because you have cancer floating around in your system and
you can't detect it and you should therefore continue to have this
treatment." But the more I studied cancer and I learned, we all
have cancer floating in our system and it is because of a good
functioning immune system that gets rid of it unless you get a
massive infusion of chemical intervention in your body, which
will disrupt the way your body functions chemically. You are going
to be all right if your immune system is strong, so I am not sure
today, quite frankly, if I would have gone through chemo. I still
have the side effects. My fingers, even after years, are still numb,
the bottoms of my feet feel like I'm walking on pebbles, so I have
lost some of the feeling in some of the nerve endings. There is a
name for it, it's called, neuropathy and I was told that the strength
of the pharmaceuticals in CHEMO literally pushes heavy metals
to your extremities.

I had asked my oncologist what I should do for myself and he
said, "You know, I am a scientist and I won't recommend anything
that isn't scientifically proven." So I said, "Okay, what should I
do for myself?" This was after having done about 50 things for
ten weeks or so anyway. He said, "Follow the Canadian Food
Guide and when you get tired, rest." So I thought, "Well, okay, I

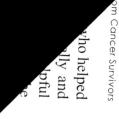

mean, you shouldn't expend all your energy, at energy to fight cancer," but I said, "Well,)asis for the Canadian Food Guide?" He said, at the nutritionists and dieticians always seem lid, "I have been scanning the literature and ıl in recommending getting off eating dairy products." This research needs to be developed further, the value of dairy for full grown adults, that is. I keep learning many new things. For example, your immune system needs certain vitamins and minerals. In particular it needs four: magnesium, sodium, potassium, and calcium. Those four ingredients are all in wheat grass or barley grass, so I have started taking wheat grass. You cannot get cancer if your immune system is strong.

I think it is really important to say, "This is MY healing process and no one else's". I went around and I spoke to a lot of cancer patients when I was having chemo, and I asked a lot of them, "What did your doctor recommend that you do for yourself?" Very rarely, was it, "Well, you might try this or you might look at that." So my learning was, if you don't change what you are doing somehow, then why do you think you won't get it again? What is the underlying cause? So, research shows this by the way too, that attitude is very often important. Those patients who say "don't bother me, I am taking off time from work, I am going to my apartment, I will get in touch with you and tell nobody to call", those are often the first people to pass on, not only with cancer, but having any disease. In speaking with the President of the Civic Hospital I mentioned this and he said, "You know Richard, somebody with a positive attitude will heal more quickly and they will survive longer." The spirit and the attitude, is absolutely fundamental. We see that with the young Senators hockey players. They break a leg and are told they will be out for 12 to 16 weeks and they are back in 8 to 10 weeks because they want to play so badly.

I am alright now. I take my vitamins and minerals and omega oils, these are all vitamins and minerals, these are not pharmaceuticals, and I have addressed what may not have been working to keep my immune system strong. The final thing I would say is that it is a heck of a journey. I am learning a lot. I would like to think that perhaps there is a reason for everything and if there is, and I can share my experience with others, then I am very happy to be able to do so.

When talking with other cancer patients, I always say, "First of all, I am not a medical doctor," so I don't comment on medical concerns. I just suggest that, "From my learning, there are many things that people can do for themselves, that are important to consider and here is what I did. You may want to do something else, but there are many, many different things I could have done as well, so it is an exciting exploration of what is available to you." I guess the message to the medical system is that as we always say, we have to look at the whole person and more and more that is coming out to bare truth in every dimension.

I make sure I drink green tea at least twice a day. I think it is wise to drink a lot of liquids anyway. Fruit is very important. It is the first thing I eat in the morning and nothing else because it is the quickest source of brain food and it goes through you within 15 or 20 minutes. It gives you power energy and it is a good cleanser as well. Following that you may want to add tea or toast or whatever. I think fresh fruits and vegetables are probably the corner stone of a good diet.

The Federal Government had a major study on health foods and natural medicines and there were 53 recommendations that were made to Allan Rock, the former Federal Minister of Health and he accepted them all. I can't track it day in and day out, but I do understand that there is hope for some of these health products. 52% of the general public utilizes complimentary medicines now in North America, so slowly, the medical schools are beginning to add these courses to look at diet and nutrition. For example, in Germany, a doctor may prescribe St. John's Wort for a mild form of depression, before prescribing Prozac. If that doesn't work, then perhaps they would propose Prozac, but they would be obliged to try the herbal treatment first. They get training with herbal medicine a lot more in Europe than we do here. We are quite, in my opinion, backward on that side of things and pretty narrow within our medical model.

It is now seven years since I contracted cancer. I was one of the growing numbers of cancer survivors. I never missed a day of work throughout my ordeal, which is not easy in public life at the best of times. I willed myself to be positive and future oriented. A special thanks to my wife Penny and my family, my friends, the Cancer Centre, naturopaths, my present oncologist Dr. Lacroix, (who is one of the most open-minded and compassionate Doctors I know) the aboriginal community and Bill O'Neil from ISM for providing me with the customized vitamins, minerals and omega oils to keep my immune system strong. And I must not forget to mention the good care and attention given me from the Cancer Centre social workers and counselors.

William Heslop

Ottawa, Ontario

___■___

The Curse That Was Within Me

When changes happened in my fife,
I took them all in stride.
My inner strength would see me through,
and my faith would be my guide.

When they said that I had cancer,
I was stunned.... could this be true?
My wife though tearful, softly said,
«our kids will help us through.»

It was a troubled time indeed
but I made a clear resolve.
Be positive and look ahead
and good things will evolve.

Warm support has been forthcoming.
Everyone has been so kind.
Despite the trauma we've been through,
it gave us peace of mind.

 The cursed tumour was removed,
the surgeon got it all.
He and the staff of nurses
performed beyond the call.

Chemo is now behind me,
it was my toughest task.
Recovery is the goal at hand
A lasting cure is all I ask

My Will To Live Is Strong

My life was going very well,
'til cancer took me down.
When I first heard that dreaded word
I vowed to "turn this thing around."

Then chemo followed surgery,
a treatment new to me.
A nurse named Jane looked for a vein
and began the therapy.

A lasting cure is imminent.
Giant gains are made each day.
When I began to worry, I reacted in a hurry,
early detection is the most effective way.

My inner strength was aggressive,
I was positive from the start.
The health care crew knew what to do,
they all gave from the heart.

The bounce is in my step once more.
My will to live is strong.
My material wealth is my new-found health,
now I'm back where I belong.

I count my blessings every day.
It was a tense and gruelling ride.
He looked after me - and made sure to see,
my loved ones were by my side

References

INTRODUCTION

■

The American Cancer Society estimates that 1,437,180 new cases of cancer and 565,650 deaths will occur in the U.S. in 2008[2]. The following table gives a list of common cancer types, including the estimated new cases and deaths in recent years in USA and Canada..

Cancer Type	Estimated New Cases USA	Estimated New Cases Canada	Estimated Deaths USA	Estimated Deaths Canada
Bladder	67,160	6,600	13,750	1,750
Breast (Female)	178,480	22,500	40,460	5,400
Colon and Rectal	153,760	20,800	52,180	8,700
Endometrial	39,080	4,100	7,400	740
Esophageal	15,560	1,300	13,940	1,300
Kidney (Renal Cell)	43,512	4,900	10,957	1,650
Leukemia	44,240	4,200	21,790	2,400
Lung	213,380	23,300	160,390	19,900
Melanoma	59,940	4,600	8,110	900
Pancreatic	37,170	3,600	33,370	3,600
Prostate	218,890	22,300	27,050	4,300
Skin (Non-melanoma)	>1,000,000	69,000	<2,000	
Thyroid	33,550	3,700	1,530	170

---

[2] http://www.cancer.org/downloads/STT/2008CAFFfinalsecured.pdf

The total number of persons diagnosed with cancer in the U.S. is approximately 10 million[3]. The Canadian Cancer Society estimates that 166,400 new cases of cancer and 73,800 deaths will occur in Canada in 2008[4]. The total number of persons living with cancer in Canada is estimated to be over 830,000[5]

When the body's cells become abnormal and duplicate out of control a tumor is formed, which may be cancerous (spreading) or benign (not spreading). Normal body cells divide in a controlled and relatively slow rate. In malignant cells the duplication is uncontrolled and often at a very rapid rate. If the tumor (also referred to as a growth) is malignant the disease may develop in other parts of the body where secondary tumors may form. Cancer is not a single disease but a wide range of different diseases. Cancers can be classified into two broad types: **haematological** (malignancies of the blood) or **solid tumors**. The name of the cancer depends on the type of tissue and/or site it develops in[6].

[3] http://fmb.cancer.gov/statistics/C-10.pdf

[4] http://www.cancer.ca/ccs/internet/standard/0,3182,3172_12851__langId-en,00.htm

[5] http://www.statcan.ca/english/freepub/84-601-XIE/2005001/incidence.htm

[6] http://www.cancerindex.org/clinks14.htm

CANCER OF THE BLADDER

Description

The bladder is in the lower part of the abdomen. It is a hollow, muscular, balloon-like organ that collects and stores urine which consists of water and waste products.

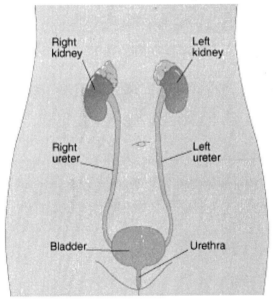

The bladder is lined with a urine-proof membrane which stops the urine being absorbed back into the body.

The kidneys produce urine, which is carried to the bladder by two tubes. The bladder then stores the urine and when it is full, the muscle of the bladder contracts, forcing the urine out of the body through a tube called the urethra.[7]

---

[7] http://www.cancerbackup.org.uk/Cancertype/Bladder/General/Thebladde

Normally in our body, cells grow and divide to form new cells. When cells grow old and die, new cells take their place. However, sometimes this process goes wrong and new cells form when the body does not need them, and old cells do not die when they should. These extra cells can form a mass of tissue called tumor.

Tumors in the bladder can be benign or malignant. Benign tumors are not cancerous and they can be removed. Malignant tumors on the other hand are cancerous. Cancer cells invade and damage nearby tissues and organs. Also, cancer cells can break away from a malignant tumor and enter the bloodstream. That is how cancer cells spread from the original tumor to form new tumors in other organs.[8]

Symptoms

The symptoms for bladder cancer are not specific. Many other diseases involving the bladder and kidney may cause similar symptoms. However, since early detection is important in curing bladder cancer, if you have the following symptoms, you should bring them to the attention of your doctor.[9]

The most common symptom of bladder cancer is blood in the urine which may be visible to the eye or may be present microscopically. This may come and go and is often painless. Sometimes blood clots may form and cause pain or obstruction to the flow of urine. Other symptoms include: a burning feeling when passing urine, a need to pass urine frequently, and pain in the pelvis[10].

---

[8] http://www.medicinenet.com/bladder_cancer/article.htm

[9] http://pathology2.jhu.edu/bladder_cancer/Symptoms.cfm

[10] http://hcd2.bupa.co.uk/fact_sheets/html/bladder_tumours.html

BREAST CANCER

———— ■ ————

Description

Like all parts of the body, the cells in the breasts usually grow and then rest in cycles. The periods of growth and rest in each cell are controlled by genes in the cell's nucleus. When genes are in good working order, they keep cell growth under control. But when genes develop an abnormality, they sometimes lose their ability to control the cycle of cell growth and rest. Breast cancer is an uncontrolled growth of breast cells. Cancer has the potential to break through normal breast tissue barriers and spread to other parts of the body. While cancer is always caused by a genetic "abnormality" only 5–10% of cancers are inherited. Instead, 90% of breast cancers are due to genetic abnormalities that happen as a result of the aging process and life in general.[11]

Breast cancer is the most common type of cancer among women, the risk of breast cancer increases with age. It is most common after the age of 50. Each breast has 15-20 sections (lobes), each of which has many smaller sections (lobules). The lobes and lobules are connected by thin tubes (ducts). The most frequent type of breast cancer is that starting in the ducts, other types include cancer beginning in the lobes or lobules, less common is inflammatory breast cancer which causes the breast to be red, and swollen[12].

———————————

[11] http://www.breastcancer.org/cmn_und_idx.html

[12] http://www.cancerindex.org/clinks3.htm

Structure of breast is illustrated by the following diagram.[13]

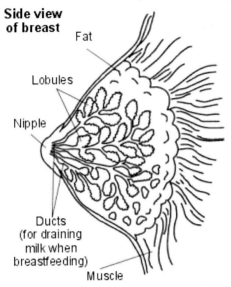

Side view of breast

Fat

Lobules

Nipple

Ducts
(for draining
milk when
breastfeeding)

Muscle

Symptoms

Cancer can occur anywhere in the breast area. It is usually noticed by any one of the following changes[14]:

- Any new lumps or old ones that change or increase in size should be checked by a doctor.
- Lump or mass in the armpit.
- A discharge from the nipple area such as bleeding or weeping.
- Hardening of the skin in the nipple area.
- Changes in the areola (the dark area around the nipple).
- Puckering of the skin in the breast area: a lemon peel effect that may appear similar to cellulite.

---

[13] http://www.patient.co.uk/showdoc/27000575/

[14] http://www.eurohealth.ie/cancom/bcan1.htm

- Inversion of the nipple such as turning inward, or at an unusual angle.

- Swelling of the upper arm or armpit just above the breast.

- Dimples.

- Breast discomfort on one side only.

- Breast pain.

- Weight loss.

- Bone pain.

- Breast enlargement on one side only.

- Change in sensation of the nipple, such as itching.

COLON AND RECTAL CANCER

Description

Colorectal cancer, also called colon cancer or bowel cancer, includes cancerous growths in the **colon, rectum** and appendix. It is the third most common form of cancer and the second leading cause of death among cancers in the Western world. Many colorectal cancers are thought to arise from **adenomatous polyps** in the colon. These mushroom-like growths are usually benign, but some may develop into cancer over time. The majority of the time, the diagnosis of localized colon cancer is through colonoscopy[15].

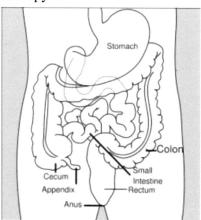

Above is a picture of the stomach and rectum[16]

[15] http://en.wikipedia.org/wiki/Colon_cancer

[16] http://en.wikipedia.org/wiki/Image:Stomach_colon_rectum_diagram.svg

Symptoms

Symptoms of colon cancer are numerous and non-specific. They include fatigue, weakness, shortness of breath, change in bowel habits, narrow stools, diarrhea or constipation, red or dark blood in stool, weight loss, abdominal pain, cramps, or bloating. Colon cancer can be present for several years before symptoms develop. Symptoms vary according to where in the large bowel the tumor is located[17].

---

[17] http://www.medicinenet.com/colon_cancer/page3.htm

ENDOMETRIAL CANCER

Description

The wall of the uterus is comprised of an inner lining (endometrium) and an outer layer of muscle tissue (myometrium).[18] Endometrial cancer is a malignancy of the endometrium (the inner lining of the uterus, or womb) and is the most common gynaecological cancer, and accounts for 13% of all cancers in women[19]

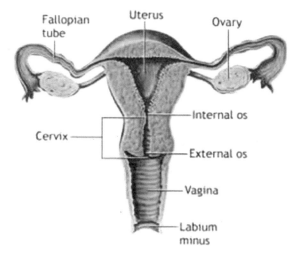

The above diagram illustrates female reproductive system.[20]

---

[18] http://www.oncologychannel.com/endometrialcancer/

[19] http://www.cancerindex.org/clinks3e.htm

[20] http://medicineworld.org/news/uterinenews.html

Symptoms

Symptoms of endometrial cancer are considered to be the following:[21]

- Chronic pelvic pain.
- In pre-menopausal women, erratic periods or bleeding between may occur.
- In post-menopausal women, any post-menopausal bleeding. This can appear as a watery, blood-soaked discharge. In 85% of cases, this bleeding is not due to cancer but from vaginal dryness due to menopausal changes.
- Pain during sex.
- Continuous feeling of tiredness.
- Painful urination or bowel movements during periods.
- Low resistance to infections.
- In women over the age of forty, extremely long, heavy or frequent episodes of bleeding

---

[21] http://www.eurohealth.ie/cancom/endocan.htm

ESOPHAGEAL CANCER

Description

The esophagus is the hollow, muscular tube that carries food and liquids from the throat to the stomach. It is part of the digestive system and is located between the windpipe (trachea) and the spine. In adults, the esophagus is about 10 inches long. Esophageal cancer usually originates in the lining of the esophagus (called the mucosa) and can develop in the upper, middle, or lower section of the organ.

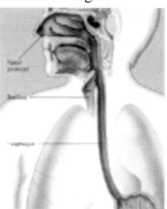

The most common types of esophageal cancer are **squamous cell carcinoma** and **adenocarcinoma**. Squamous cell carcinoma develops in flat cells that line the esophagus. Approximately 60% of squamous cell carcinomas develop in the middle third of the organ, 30% occur in the lower third, and 10% occur in the upper third.

Adenocarcinoma develops in the lining of the esophagus and is associated with a condition called **Barrett's esophagus**. This type usually occurs in the lower third of the esophagus[22].

Symptoms

Early cancer of the esophagus usually does not cause symptoms. In as many as 50% of cases, the disease is locally advanced or has already spread at the time of diagnosis. Symptoms of the disease include the following:

- Coughing up blood
- Difficulty swallowing (dysphagia) or painful swallowing (odynophagia)
- Hoarseness or chronic cough
- Iron-deficiency anemia (may be diagnosed through a blood test)
- Pain in the throat, back, behind the breastbone (sternum), or between the shoulder blades
- Severe weight loss
- Vomiting[23]

---

[22] http://www.oncologychannel.com/esophagealcancer/index.shtm

[23] http://www.oncologychannel.com/esophagealcancer/riskfactors.shtml#symptoms

KIDNEY CANCER

Description

The kidneys are the primary organs of the urinary system. The kidneys are the organs that filter the blood, remove the wastes, and excrete the wastes in the urine. They are the organs that perform the functions of the urinary system. The other components are accessory structures to eliminate the urine from the body. The paired kidneys are located between the twelfth thoracic and third lumbar vertebrae, one on each side of the vertebral column.[24]

Frontal section through the Kidney

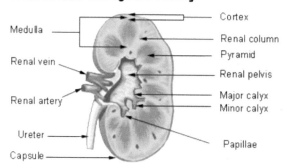

Kidney cancer forms in tissues of the kidneys and it includes renal cell carcinoma, i.e., cancer that forms in the lining of very small tubes in the kidney that filter the blood and remove waste products and renal pelvis carcinoma. i.e., cancer that forms in the centre of the kidney where urine collects.[25]

---

[24] http://training.seer.cancer.gov/module_anatomy/unit11_2_uri_comp1_kidney.html

[25] http://www.cancer.gov/cancertopics/types/kidney

Renal cell carcinoma (RCC), the most common form, accounts for approximately 85% of all cases. In RCC, cancerous (malignant) cells develop in the lining of the kidney's tubules and grow into a mass called a tumor. In most cases, a single tumor develops, although more than one tumor can develop within one or both kidneys.[26]

Symptoms

In its early stages, kidney cancer usually causes no obvious signs or troublesome symptoms. However, as a kidney tumor grows, symptoms may occur. These may include:

- Blood in the urine. Blood may be present one day and not the next. In some cases, a person can actually see the blood, or traces of it may be found in *urinalysis*, a lab test often performed as part of a regular medical checkup.

- A lump or mass in the kidney area.

Other less common kidney cancer symptoms may include:

- Fatigue;
- Loss of appetite;
- Weight loss;
- Recurrent fevers;
- A pain in the side that doesn't go away; and/or
- A general feeling of poor health[27]

---

[26] http://www.urologychannel.com/kidneycancer/ .

[27] http://www.healthnewsflash.com/conditions/kidney_cancer.htm#5

LEUKEMIA

Description

L eukemia is a malignant disease (cancer) of the bone marrow and blood. It is characterized by the uncontrolled accumulation of blood cells. Leukemia is divided into four categories:

- Acute Lymphocytic Leukemia
- Chronic Lymphocytic Leukemia
- Acute Myelogenous Leukemia
- Chronic Myelogenous Leukemia

Acute leukemia is a rapidly progressing disease that results in the accumulation of immature, functionless cells in the marrow and blood. The marrow often can no longer produce enough normal red blood cells, white blood cells and platelets. Anemia, a deficiency of red cells, develops in virtually all leukemia patients. The lack of normal white cells impairs the body's ability to fight infections. A shortage of platelets results in bruising and easy bleeding. Chronic leukemia progresses more slowly and allows greater numbers of more mature, functional cells to be made.[28]

Microscopic views of normal and abnormal bone marrow and sectioned blood vessel demonstrating blood cells flowing inside are illustrated below.[29]

---

[28] http://www.leukemia-lymphoma.org/all_page?item_id=9346
[29] http://www.fotosearch.com/LIF145/pdb02010/

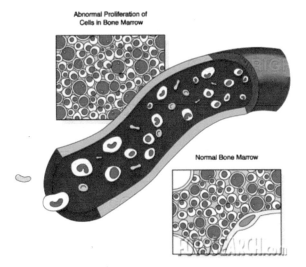

Abnormal Proliferation of
Cells in Bone Marrow

Normal Bone Marrow

Blood cells are illustrated by the following diagram.[30]

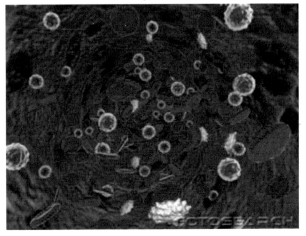

30 http://www.fotosearch.com/PSK125/1574r-018972/

Symptoms

The first indications of leukemia often are nonspecific. They may occur with other cancerous as well as non-cancerous disorders. Although signs and symptoms vary for each type of leukemia, there are some general features. Broad symptoms of leukemia may include:

- Fatigue
- Malaise (vague feeling of bodily discomfort)
- Abnormal bleeding
- Excessive bruising
- Weakness
- Reduced exercise tolerance
- Weight loss
- Bone or joint pain
- Infection and fever
- Abdominal pain or "fullness"
- Enlarged spleen, lymph nodes, and liver

LUNG CANCER

Description

The lung is the essential respiration organ in air-breathing vertebrates. Its principal function is to transport oxygen from the atmosphere into the bloodstream, and to excrete carbon dioxide from the bloodstream into the atmosphere. This exchange of gases is accomplished in the mosaic of specialized cells that form millions of tiny, exceptionally thin-walled air sacs called alveoli. The lungs also have non-respiratory functions such as gas exchange and regulation of **hydrogen ion concentration.**[31]

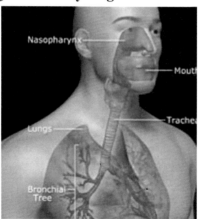

Cancer of the lung, like all cancers, results from an abnormality in the body's basic unit of life, the cell. Normally, the body maintains a system of checks and balances on cell growth so that cells divide to produce new cells only when needed. Disruption

---

[31] http://en.wikipedia.org/wiki/Lung

of this system of checks and balances on cell growth results in an uncontrolled division and proliferation of cells that eventually forms a mass known as a tumor.[32]

Symptoms

One fourth of all people with lung cancer have no symptoms when the cancer is diagnosed. These cancers are usually identified incidentally when a chest x-ray is performed for another reason. The other three fourths of people develop some symptoms. The symptoms are due to direct effects of the primary tumor; to effects of metastatic tumors in other parts of the body; or to malignant disturbances of hormones, blood, or other systems.

Symptoms of primary lung cancers include cough, coughing up blood, chest pain, and shortness of breath.

- A new cough in a smoker or a former smoker should raise concern for lung cancer.

- A cough that does not go away or gets worse over time should be evaluated by a doctor.

- Coughing up blood occurs in a significant number of people who have lung cancer.

- Chest pain is a symptom in about one fourth of people with lung cancer. The pain is dull, aching, and persistent and may involve other structures surrounding the lung.

- Wheezing or hoarseness may signal blockage or inflammation in the lungs that may go along with cancer.

- Repeated respiratory infections, such as bronchitis or pneumonia, can be a sign of lung cancer.

- Shortness of breath usually results from a blockage in part of the lung, collection of fluid around the lung (pleural effusion), or the spread of tumor through the lungs.[33]

---

[32] http://www.medicinenet.com/lung_cancer/article.htm

[33] http://www.emedicinehealth.com/lung_cancer/page3_em.htm

MELANOMA

—————■—————

Description

Melanoma is a malignant tumor of melanocytes which are found predominantly in skin but also in the bowel and the eye. It is one of the rarer types of skin cancer but causes the majority of skin cancer related deaths. Melanocytes are cells located in the bottom layer, the basal lamina, of the skin's epidermis and in the middle layer of the eye, the uvea[34].

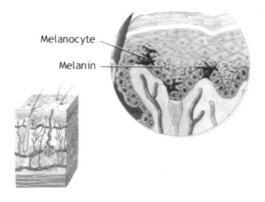

Melanocyte

Melanin

Melanoma develops in the cells that produce melanin, the pigment that gives your skin its color. Melanoma can also form in the eyes and, rarely, in internal organs, such as the intestines. Although melanomas make up the smallest percentage of all skin cancers, they cause the greatest number of deaths, because they're more likely to spread to different parts of the body. The exact cause of all melanomas is not clear, but exposure to ultraviolet (UV)

[34] http://en.wikipedia.org/wiki/Melanoma

radiation from sunlight or tanning lamps and beds greatly increases the risk of developing melanoma. Knowing the warning signs of skin cancer can help ensure that cancerous changes are detected and treated before they have a chance to spread. Melanoma can be successfully treated if you catch it early.[35]

Symptoms

Melanoma may be formed from an existing mole or freckle, or begin to grow from a normal-appearing area of the skin. Any change in a mole's appearance or the growth of a new mole may be a sign of skin cancer. Suspicious moles or freckles should be checked by a doctor.

Melanomas vs. normal moles:

- Moles and freckles usually are brown or black and have a defined edge or border.

- Melanomas are usually multi-colored and may combine different shades of brown and black, sometimes with areas of red, blue, or white. They often have an irregular or uneven border.

Melanomas often show the following symptoms:

- **A**symmetry, when one half of the growth has a different shape than the other.

- **B**order irregular, when the growth has scalloped or uneven edges.

- **C**olor varied, when the growth is more than one color. Melanomas may be black, shades of brown and tan, and even have specks of red, white, and blue.

- **D**iameter, when the size, measured edge to edge, is bigger than the diameter of a pencil eraser.[36]

---

[35] http://www.mayoclinic.com/health/melanoma/DS00439

[36] http://www.ehealthmd.com/library/melanoma/MEL_symptoms.html

NON-HODGKIN'S and HODGKIN'S LYMPHOMA

———————■———————

Description

The lymph system is part of the immune system and is made up of the following:

- Lymph: Colorless, watery fluid that travels through the lymph system and carries white blood cells called lymphocytes. Lymphocytes protect the body against infections and the growth of tumors.

- Lymph vessels: A network of thin tubes that collect lymph from different parts of the body and return it to the bloodstream.

- Lymph nodes: Small, bean-shaped structures that filter lymph and store white blood cells that help fight infection and disease. Lymph nodes are located along the network of lymph vessels found throughout the body. Clusters of lymph nodes are found in the underarm, pelvis, neck, abdomen, and groin.

- Spleen: An organ that makes lymphocytes, filters the blood, stores blood cells, and destroys old blood cells. It is on the left side of the abdomen near the stomach.

- Thymus: An organ in which lymphocytes grow and multiply. The thymus is in the chest behind the breastbone.

- Tonsils: Two small masses of lymph tissue at the back of the throat. The tonsils make lymphocytes.

- Bone marrow: The soft, spongy tissue in the center of large bones. Bone marrow makes white blood cells, red blood cells, and platelets.

Lymphomas are divided into two general types: Hodgkin lymphoma and non-Hodgkin lymphoma.

Non-Hodgkin lymphomas can occur at any age and are often marked by enlarged lymph nodes, fever, and weight loss. There are many different types of non-Hodgkin lymphoma, which can be divided into aggressive (fast-growing) and indolent (slow-growing) types and can be classified as either B-cell or T-cell non-Hodgkin lymphoma. B-cell non-Hodgkin lymphomas include Burkitt lymphoma, diffuse large B-cell lymphoma, follicular lymphoma, immunoblastic large cell lymphoma, precursor B-lymphoblastic lymphoma, and mantle cell lymphoma. T-cell non-Hodgkin lymphomas include mycosis fungoides, anaplastic large cell lymphoma, and precursor T-lymphoblastic lymphoma. Lymphomas related to lymphoproliferative disorders following bone marrow or stem cell transplantation are usually B-cell non-Hodgkin lymphomas. Prognosis and treatment depend on the stage and type of disease.[37]

---

[37] http://www.cancer.gov/cancertopics/pdq/treatment/adult-non-hodgkins/patien

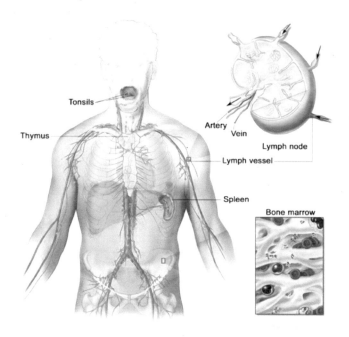

There are two main types of Hodgkin lymphoma: classical and nodular lymphocyte-predominant. Most Hodgkin lymphomas are the classical type. The classical type is broken down into the following four subtypes:

- Nodular sclerosing Hodgkin lymphoma.
- Mixed cellularity Hodgkin lymphoma.
- Lymphocyte depletion Hodgkin lymphoma.
- Lymphocyte-rich classical Hodgkin lymphoma.

Symptoms

Symptoms of NHL may appear suddenly or may develop gradually over a long period of time and can occur in many places and in many forms, some of which produce no symptoms at all. About two-thirds of adults diagnosed with non-Hodgkin's lymphoma (NHL) notice swollen, painless lymph nodes in the armpit, groin, near the collarbone, or in some area of the neck, including the back of the neck. Sometimes a node may rupture and weep.[38]

Because lymph tissue is found throughout the body, Hodgkin lymphoma can begin in almost any part of the body and spread to almost any tissue or organ in the body. Symptoms of Hodgkin's disease may include the following:

- A painless swelling in the lymph nodes in the neck, underarm, or groin
- Unexplained recurrent fevers
- Night sweats
- Unexplained weight loss
- Itchy skin

When symptoms like these occur, they are not sure signs of Hodgkin's disease. In most cases, they are actually caused by other, less serious conditions, such as the flu. When symptoms like these persist, however, it is important to see a doctor so that any illness can be diagnosed and treated. Only a doctor can make a diagnosis of Hodgkin's disease. Do not wait to feel pain; early Hodgkin's disease may not cause pain.[39]

---

[38] http://www.patientcenters.com/lymphoma/news/nhl1.html#symptoms

[39] http://www.healthnewsflash.com/conditions/hodgkins_cancer.htm#2

PANCREATIC CANCER

Description

Pancreatic cancer is one of the most serious of cancers. It develops when cancerous cells form in the tissues of your pancreas, i.e., a large organ that lies horizontally behind the lower part of the stomach. Pancreas secretes enzymes that aid digestion and hormones that help regulate the metabolism of carbohydrates. Pancreatic cancer spreads rapidly and is seldom detected in its early stages, which is a major reason why it's a leading cause of cancer death. Signs and symptoms may not appear until the disease is quite advanced. By that time, the cancer is likely to have spread to other parts of the body and surgical removal may not be possible.[40]

The location of Pancreas illustrated by the following diagram.[41]

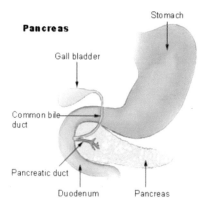

[40] http://www.mayoclinic.com/health/pancreatic-cancer/DS00357
[41] http://upload.wikimedia.org/wikipedia/commons/6/64/Illu_pancrease.jpg

Symptoms

It is rather difficult to diagnose pancreatic cancer as the pancreas is so deep within the body and symptoms vary depending on the location of the tumour in the pancreas and which cells or function of the pancreas is affected by the tumour. The symptoms of pancreatic cancer can also be quite vague and non specific, i.e., may be caused by many other more common and less serious conditions. Diagnosis can be delayed as the medical doctor tries to rule out other causes such as hepatitis, gall stones, irritable bowel syndrome and stress. For example jaundice can be an early sign of a tumour in the head of the pancreas affecting the bile duct and back pain can be a late sign of a tumour in the body or tail of the pancreas possibly affecting the nerves and spine. Symptoms may include:

- General discomfort or pain around the stomach area
- Sickness
- Bowel disturbances
- Diabetes
- Jaundice
- Skin itching
- Loss of appetite
- Unexplained weight loss
- Back pain
- Low mood and depression[42]

---

[42] http://www.pancreaticcancer.org.uk/PCSymptoms.htm

PROSTATE CANCER

———■———

Description

T he prostate gland is located in the pelvis, below the bladder, above the urethral sphincter and the penis, and in front of the rectum in men. The gland is covered by a membrane (called the prostate capsule) that produces prostate-specific antigen.[43] The prostate produces the fluid that mixes with sperm when a man ejaculates.[44]

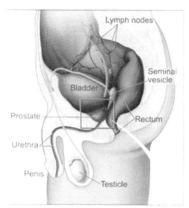
This shows the prostate and nearby organs.

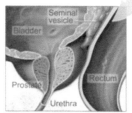
This shows the inside of the prostate, urethra, rectum, and bladder.

---

[43] http://www.urologychannel.com/prostatecancer/index.shtml
[44] http://www.aicr.org.uk/ProstateFAQs.stm?source=Adwords

Prostate cancer is a disease in which cancer develops in the prostate. Cancer occurs when cells of the prostate mutate and begin to multiply out of control. These cells may spread from the prostate to other parts of the body, especially the bones and lymph nodes. Prostate cancer may cause pain, difficulty in urinating, erectile dysfunction and other symptoms.[45]

Symptoms

The main symptoms include difficulty passing urine, inability to urinate, passing urine often (particularly at night), weak or interrupted urine flow, pain when urinating, blood in the urine and pain in the lower back, hips and upper thighs. However, all of these symptoms can also be caused by other conditions such as benign prostate enlargement.[46]

---

[45] http://en.wikipedia.org/wiki/Prostate_cancer
[46] http://www.aicr.org.uk/ProstateFAQs.stm?source=Adwords

SKIN CANCER

Description

The skin has two main layers:

- The **epidermis** is the top layer of the skin. It is mostly made of flat cells. These are squamous cells. Under the squamous cells in the deepest part of the epidermis are round cells called basal cells. Cells called melanocytes make the pigment (color) found in skin and are located in the lower part of the epidermis.

- The **dermis** is under the epidermis. It contains blood vessels, lymph vessels, and glands. Some of these glands make sweat, which helps cool the body. Other glands make sebum, an oily substance that helps keep the skin from drying out. Sweat and sebum reach the surface of the skin through tiny openings called pores.

This picture shows the layers of the skin.[47]

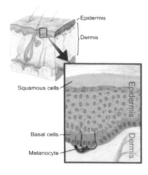

[47] http://www.cancer.gov/cancertopics/ wyntk/skin/page2

Skin cancer is a malignant growth on the skin which can have many causes. Skin cancer generally develops in the epidermis, the outermost layer of skin, so a tumor is usually clearly visible. This makes most skin cancers detectable in the early stages. There are three common types of skin cancer, each of which is named after the type of skin cell from which it arises. The most common types of skin cancer are basal cell carcinoma (BCC) and squamous cell carcinoma (SCC) which may be locally disfiguring but are unlikely to spread to other parts of the body. The most dangerous type is malignant melanoma. This form of skin cancer can be fatal if not treated early but comprises only a small proportion of all skin cancers.[48]

Symptoms

Skin cancer symptoms can be one or more of many things, including: a spot, sore, or mole with its shape, size, color, changing. Some more direct skin cancer symptoms are:

- A lump on the skin that may be small, smooth, pale, waxy, or red, and may bleed or crust over;
- A flat patch on the skin that may be red, rough, dry, or scaly
- A lump or patch that grows or changes color or shape;
- A sore that does not heal;
- An itchy lump or patch;
- A spot that becomes itchy, tender, or painful;
- A spot that becomes red and/or swollen;
- A mole that grows or otherwise changes its appearance.

Most skin cancer symptoms will usually show up on the parts of the skin that are exposed to sunlight the most, such as: the face, head, neck, arms, and hands.[49]

---

[48] http://en.wikipedia.org/wiki/Skin_cancer#Types
[49] http://www.womens-health-fitness.com/skin-cancer-symptoms.html

THYROID CANCER

Description

Thyroid cancer develops in the thyroid, a butterfly-shaped gland located at the base of your neck, just below the Adam's apple. Although the thyroid gland is small, it produces hormones that regulate every aspect of the metabolism, from heart rate to how quickly a person burns calories. Sometimes one may develop one or more solid or fluid-filled lumps called nodules in the thyroid. Most of these are non-cancerous (benign) and cause no symptoms. But a small percentage are cancerous (malignant).[50]

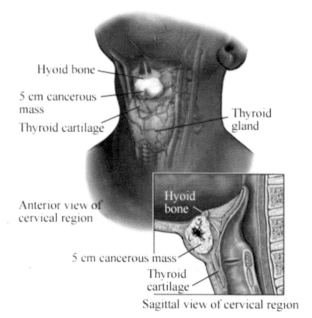

Hyoid bone

5 cm cancerous mass

Thyroid cartilage

Thyroid gland

Anterior view of cervical region

Hyoid bone

5 cm cancerous mass

Thyroid cartilage

Sagittal view of cervical region

---

[50] http://www.mayoclinic.com/health/thyroid-cancer/DS00492

There are several types of thyroid cancer, including:

- **Papillary Carcinoma** is the most common type. It usually grows very slowly, and often spreads to lymph nodes in the neck

- **Follicular Carcinoma** is the second most common type. It usually stays in the thyroid gland but can spread to other parts of the body, such as the lungs and bones. It does not usually spread to the lymph nodes.

- **Anaplastic Carcinoma** is a rare form of thyroid cancer. It quickly invades the neck and other parts of the body. .

- **Medullary Thyroid Carcinoma (MTC)** is a form of cancer that develops from cells in the thyroid gland called C-cells. It often spreads to the lymph nodes, lungs, or liver before a thyroid nodule has been discovered

- **Thyroid Lymphoma** is a rare type of thyroid cancer. Many cases occur in people who have a disease called Hashimoto's thyroiditis, in which the immune system attacks a person's own thyroid gland.[51]

Symptoms

Most commonly, thyroid cancers in the early stage produce no symptoms. As the cancer grows, a small lump or nodule can be felt in the neck. The vast majority of thyroid are caused by benign conditions, but about one per cent of these lumps represent early stages of thyroid cancer. If the cancer spreads, it can cause symptoms that include:

- Problems with swallowing

---

[51] http://images.google.ca/imgres?imgurl=http://services.epnet.com/GetImage. aspx/getImage.aspx%3FImageIID%3D4675&imgrefurl=http://healthlibrary.epnet. com/GetContent.aspx%3Ftoken%3D8482e079-8512-47c2-960c-a403c77a5e4c%26 chunkiid%3D11507&h=388&w=366&sz=22&tbnid=y3aNrK2-_QUVYM:&tbnh=1 23&tbnw=116&prev=/images%3Fq%3Dthyroid%2Bcancer%2Bpictures%26um%3 D1&start=1&sa=X&oi=images&ct=image&cd=1

- Hoarseness
- Enlarged lymph nodes in the neck
- Breathing difficulty
- Pain in the throat and/or neck

About 99% of nodules in the thyroid gland are benign, but only a doctor can determine if a lump in the neck is cancerous. Even the symptoms above can be caused by infections and other benign conditions.[52]

---

[52] http://www.medicinenet.com/script/main/art.asp?articlekey=53303

ABOUT THE
AUTHORS

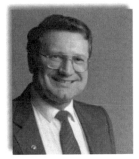

Frank Hegyi is a scientist, entrepreneur and author. He has spent over 38 years in community service. He is past District Governor of Kiwanis International. At age 66 he was diagnosed with prostate cancer. During radiation treatment, he wrote a book entitled: Dare to Take the Next Step (see www.frankhegyi.com) which contains inspirational stories about his colourful international adventures. Frank dedicated his stories of life experiences to his family who gave him strong support during the cancer treatment. He is a proud cancer survivor. He celebrated his 70th birthday with a 10K bicycle ride (on Nortel Tour) with his 5 year old grandson (Ryan) and together they raised $750 for CHEO cancer research.

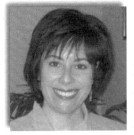

Roslyn Franken, diagnosed with cancer at age 29, fought back to become a long-term survivor. As she approached 40, Roslyn's personal struggles with food, weight and lifestyle issues led to the creation of the techniques that changed her life. By putting the principles into practice, she reached and maintains her current, healthy weight and lifestyle and remains cancer-free. Roslyn now provides Motivational Speaking and Personal Counseling services to individuals and groups wishing to change their lives for the better through weight and lifestyle management, using the principles she developed and now shares in her book The A List: 9 Guiding Principles for Healthy Eating and Positive Living. *www. roslynfranken.com*

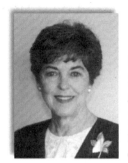

Jacquelin Holzman is a former mayor of Ottawa (1991–1997), with more than 15 years' experience in politics and over 50 years of community service. She served as chair of the Ottawa Congress Centre from 1998 to 2003, has been involved in fundraising for The Ottawa Hospital Foundation and the Ottawa Boys and Girls Club, and has served as governor of Algonquin College, the Community Foundation of Ottawa and as the Honorary Lieutenant Colonel of the Cameron Highlanders of Ottawa. A few months after leaving the mayor's office, she was diagnosed with breast cancer, and was treated successfully and became an advocate for breast cancer related causes. Jackie and her daughter have raised over $200,000 for cancer care and research at The Ottawa Hospital and the Ottawa Health Research Institute during the past 10 years.

———————■———————

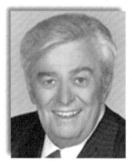

Max Keeping is VP News at CTV Ottawa, and anchor of its flagship 6pm newscast for 36 years. His community involvement has helped raise more than $100 million charitable dollars. He's received the Order of Canada, Order of Ontario, a Gemini Humanitarian Award, and an Honourary degree from the University of Ottawa. A wing of the Children's Hospital (CHEO) is named in his honour. He's a survivor of prostate cancer.

———————■———————

212 Immune system needs
sodium potassium magnesium
calcium
green tea
fruit for breakfast